BUILDING A MODERN DEMENTIA SERVICE

Roger Bullock MA, MRCPsych

Kingshill Research Centre, Avon and Wiltshire Mental Health Partnership NHS Trust, Victoria Hospital, Swindon, UK

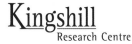

D0293704

This copy of *Building a Modern Dementia Service* is given as a service to medicine by Janssen-Cilag Ltd and Shire Pharmaceuticals Ltd. The views expressed herein are not necessarily those of Janssen-Cilag Ltd or Shire Pharmaceuticals Ltd.

ALTMAN

Published by Altman Publishing, 65 Lake View, Edgware, Middlesex, HA8 7SA, UK

First edition 2002

Typeset in 10/12 Optima by Scribe Design, Gillingham, Kent
Printed in Great Britain by George Over Ltd, Rugby

ISBN 1-86036-021-1

A catalogue record for this book is available from the British Library

∞ Printed on acid-free text paper, manufactured in accordance with ANSI/NISO Z39.48-1992 (Permanence of Paper)

CONTENTS

ABOUT THE AUTHOR

Dr Roger Bullock MA, MRCPsych is clinical lead in old age psychiatry services and Director of the Kingshill Research Centre in Swindon. The main work of the centre is research into dementia, ranging from drug development work, neuropsychology and measurement, and incorporating this into service design. His interests are in mild cognitive impairment and the effect pharmacotherapy will have on this patient group, and the effective management of the behavioural disorders seen in sufferers of dementia.

Dr Bullock has been involved in clinical trials in dementia, psychosis and depression for 10 years. He has published in the area and presented at many major conferences. Impending projects include the implementation of a published care pathway in dementia, and work on the standardisation of memory clinics. He has academic affiliation to the University of Bath, and is collaborating in research around the UK and Europe.

CONTRIBUTORS

J. Jaime Caro MDCM FRCPC FACP
Siobhan Jackson PgDip R Art Therapist
Claire Leonard MCSP
Judith O'Brien RN
Lucie Spurway BSc Speech Therapy MRCSLT
Alex Ward PhD MRPharmS
Alison Warren MSc DipCOT SROT
Oonagh Wigley MmedSci Clinical Communication Studies MRCSLT

1 INTRODUCTION

A famous story tells us of a tourist, who on becoming lost, asks a local the way. 'If I were going there, I wouldn't start from here' was the less than helpful answer. In some ways though, this bears resemblance to the position found when trying to set a strategy for modernising our current dementia services.

Current requirements needed to provide a comprehensive service for people that suffer from dementia can be divided into a set of building blocks that can be assembled to ensure a package of near total care. These blocks have evolved with the history of the way dementia has been treated, which has made strides over the last 20 years in an opportunistic and piecemeal way. It has flourished where its pioneers and enthusiasts have driven change, while in some areas it has been left to fend as a true Cinderella subject or, worse still, asset-stripped to pay for services that attracted more attention. This has left the UK with a situation where the range of spend in the individual trusts is from £5 to £235 per head of population (Audit Commission 2000), making any wish to achieve equity across the country a demanding proposition.

This means that services in the UK differ dramatically, usually not in philosophy or the 'what' they aspire to provide, but in resources. This is also often the case in Europe and beyond, where each country often has ingenious arrangements that keep the building blocks separate. The situation has been placed in sharper perspective as new treatments start to pressurise the same scant resource. To make sense of this situation, one needs to understand the historical perspective, the necessary building blocks, how to effectively assemble them within the guidance of recent government publications, and some perspectives on the organisational structures that may deliver them. To prevent a repetition of this diversity of services continuing into the future, a move towards proactive services, with a grasp on what is coming in the future, should produce enduring and flexible resources, which are patient, not service, driven.

Effectively we now have a jigsaw, often with missing pieces, which has been put together in different ways. This is because all services have started, and will currently continue to do so, from different points. The aim of this book is to define the jigsaw pieces and offer ideas on how best to assemble them, in a way tailored to local demand. In it I draw on experience from setting up the Swindon services, and the hard work the team continues to put in, and also on conversations with colleagues around the UK and beyond. This book does not give all the answers by any means, but I hope it helps create debate and a chance to move toward a common point, from where future modernisation can start, making the story this section began with less representative.

2 HISTORY

Patients with late-onset mental illnesses, especially the dementias, were admitted to a large Nightingale back ward continuing care beds in the asylums, where people spent the last years of their life in large dormitories. The availability of large numbers of beds and the absence of any treatment other than sedation and containment led to a forgotten culture with minimal therapeutic input.

Early pioneers sought to improve the quality of life for patients on these wards, and in doing so created a subspeciality interested in the mental illnesses of the elderly, dubbed psychogeriatrics. This dealt mainly with the problems of severe dementia, particularly the difficult behaviours, and was predominantly hospital based.

These services started to move to the community as institutions closed, but were still characterised by referrals late in the course of the illness, usually as the difficult behaviours became too much for the carer to cope with. At this point, the carer approached the GP. Where services existed, these patients were referred for specialist assessment and management. Thus, a few new community services started to offer services to patients with late moderate-to-severe dementia, for a period pre-institutionalisation.

- Closure of the asylums released long-stay funds, but often finance did not consistently find its way to the community. As a result, these patients lost some of their initial health investment, appropriate community services were not put in place, and the public lost trust (Trieman and Wills 1996).
- The speciality of old age psychiatry grew and assumed the mantle of treating all mental illness in the over-65 age group. This led to a shared emphasis with the functional illnesses like depression and paraphrenia and often a lesser input in to the dementing illnesses, which were diagnosed and returned to primary care for long-term management. The border with general psychiatry set a false boundary based on retirement age – an unresolved issue to this day. The increase in functional work led to dementia care sharing what resources it had obtained from psychiatry. At this stage, geriatric

medicine was referred many of the moderate cases in order to exclude treatable causes – again, the norm was to diagnose and return to the GP. This meant care became fragmented and any attempt at continuity suffered (Connell and Kole 1994).

- The Community Care Act appeared in 1990 (Department of Health 1990). This legislation pointed the way to developing better community services in mental health, and attempted to get health and social services working in a more unified manner to provide continuity of care. Old age psychiatry was now an established and growing speciality, with a developed community assessment and treatment philosophy. It did still rely on referral from primary care, so was seeing patients at the moderate-to-severe stage as the bulk of routine work.

- The cholinergic theory of the 1970s bore fruition in the late 1990s with the introduction of licensed symptomatic treatments for mild-to-moderate Alzheimer's disease. This led to two changes – increased awareness among the patients and public; and a realisation by services that they needed to cater now for mild-to-moderate patients.

- Increased user and carer involvement has continued to drive services towards providing earlier diagnosis and better information, and following the NICE (National Institute for Clinical Excellence 2001) decision, a desire to use and understand the treatments.

- Treatment for Alzheimer's disease has now changed services for dementia in a fundamental way towards a more neurological basis, bringing with it a host of training and infrastructure issues. The main responsibility for providing services for dementia now rests with old age psychiatry in the UK (neurology in Europe), but services for those with dementia remain fragmented and inefficient.

- Primary care has not kept pace with the change in dementia care, and feels lacking in the skills to help [Forget Me Not (FMN); Audit Commission 2000]. Old age psychiatry community services have evolved into sophisticated multidisciplinary teams offering complex and continuous care planning, in a situation that could be construed as 'specialist primary care'.

- The neurobiology of the dementias and the neurodegenerative diseases is slowly being understood, and along with it complex pharmacology and genetics are pointing toward treatment options. The implementation of the findings into mainstream clinical practice is falling on psychiatrists whose training is more towards social intervention, causing some disharmony, delaying the step towards mild illness.

- Other degenerative disorders, notably Parkinson's disease, have psychiatric sequelae, and are increasingly being seen by psychiatrists in their routine work, making the field move further towards neurology, and changing our training requirements.
- Mild cognitive impairment and the possibility of preventative work now position the 'early-adopting' clinics to make a further leap of faith to start developing services aimed at the minimally impaired to those with mild Alzheimer's. Future services may be looking at even earlier interventions using a public health model of primary and secondary prevention.

Pieces of the puzzle

The jigsaw puzzle emerging from the historical context has many pieces, but its main components are:

- Improving awareness, detection and referrals
- Streamlining the assessment process
- Better utilisation of staff
- Gearing up to increasing treatment paradigms
- Putting the right components in the correct juxtaposition
- Questioning old practice
- Moving away from the medical model in some areas, while creating it in others, that is, developing the appropriate role for doctors in the dementia pathway
- Managing significant change and empowering staff during the process
- Having clear principles and development goals
- Imagining what the future may hold and creating the flexibility to address it.

This book follows this route in a way that discusses the pieces and their relevance, and offers practical steps in their implementation. The content is to stimulate discussion and local ideas, not dictate the how.

A recent publication, *An Integrated Care Pathway for Dementia* (Naidoo and Bullock 2001) attempts to summarise secondary evidence in a format that matches progression through the disease. In it dementia is divided into various progressive stages in order to structure the evidence. This is in many ways a complementary piece of work, citing the evidence base for much of what this volume proposes. This and other publications (Bannerjee and Dickinson 1997) show that much of what we do has a reasonable base in fact, while also indicating where more information is needed.

3 DETECTION AND REFERRAL

Historically we have evolved services backwards through the illness, adding expertise and increasing specialism as we go. The problem now is that the diagnostic expertise is needed at the early presenting stage of the illness, where up to 50% of general practitioners (Audit Commission 2000) feel least confident in what they are seeing, raising the issue of their training (Connell and Kole 1994; de Lepeleire and Heyrman 1994). Worse, 50% feel that nothing can be offered anyway (Audit Commission 2000). As a result, education in primary care and targeting of low referring practices to help detect and refer patients must be a key priority, and both were recommendations in the Forget me Not document (Audit Commission 2000). Intervention programmes have been devised and are under evaluation (Iliffe 1994; Iliffe *et al.* 1998). Figure 3.1 shows why further work is needed. It is a schematic model of what happens in Alzheimer's disease (AD), with a line marked to show the average position where GPs refer. This was derived from workshops involving 138 GPs who indicated on a scale the point they

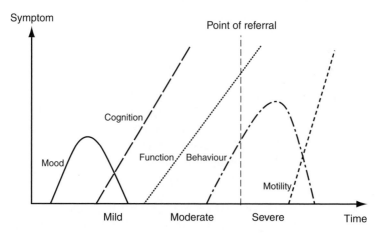

Figure 3.1 Point of referral in Alzheimer's disease

usually refer patients. This point occurs after cognition has been lost, function is grossly impaired and behaviour has pushed the carer to the brink. In physics, Hooke's law describes how a spring bounces back when stretched, until it finally stretches beyond its limit and never recovers. This is a useful paradigm for imagining carers, who behave similarly. Starting services from here misses a wealth of treatment opportunity and is focusing most of the resource at a limited part of the disease process. It is about managing the carers through this phase, having little to do with the patients and their needs.

Unfortunately, a survey of UK consultants carried out by our department in January 2001 bore out the biased position towards more advanced dementia. It showed that 25% of AD work was on mild dementia, 40% on moderate and 35% on severe. This is a baseline that needs to shift towards the mild spectrum and hopefully the NICE guidance will contribute towards this.

The premise that I have set up implies that the early diagnosis of dementia, particularly AD, is both desirable and necessary, and the focus of the book is about moving towards this goal. No controlled studies prove this assumption, but the following statements support it:

- Patients and carers want to understand their illnesses more and be given the diagnosis early enough to make choices (Askham 1995; McCurry and Teri 1997).
- Patients and carers want to reverse the feeling of disempowerment that has been the impression to date (McWilliam 1994) and even though old, be included in decision making and treatment opportunity (Harding, 1997).
- The presence of effective symptomatic treatments requires their use when symptoms are minimal.
- A move towards disease modification and prevention of decline is already underway. Brookmeyer (Brookmeyer *et al.* 1998; Brookmeyer and Gray 2000) has predicted that a 1-year delay in progression in AD could reduce the prevalence of severe dementia by 20%, and a 2-year delay could lead to a 50% fall. The impact of this would be profound, both financially (Wimo *et al.* 1994) and emotionally.
- Our understanding of normal and abnormal cognitive ageing is improving (Ritchie 1998) and so the information and treatments we can provide improve with it.

- Commissioners must soon start to question how current services continue to be justified, but without a coordinated model may rely too much on the belief that much of what needs to be provided could be done by primary care.

Detection

For many patients presenting to a GP, the symptoms they describe fit a learned pattern that provokes a response. This happens less in those with dementia, which, allied with the belief that cognitive impairment is inevitable, makes detection less likely. Also, patients may not present themselves (Grace 1994). The first contact with the GP sets the whole future pattern of care for a person with dementia (McIntosh *et al.* 1997). All dementia services have to assist in making this contact a positive event, so that more patients gain access to treatment opportunities. Figure 3.2 shows the extent of the problem in the UK with

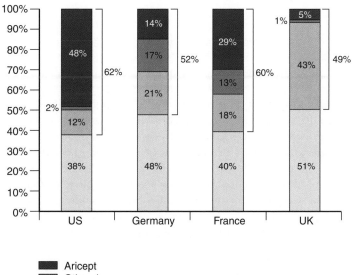

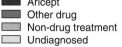

Figure 3.2 Alzheimer's disease population diagnosed and treated, 1999

51% of the existing patients undiagnosed, and only an eighth of those that are receiving cholinesterase therapy. What is needed is the creation of an accepted pattern that triggers a better assessment. As depression is often a comorbid factor in early dementias, along with problems in executive function, then patients who come to the GP with loss of memory, feeling low or less able, confused or lacking in confidence, should have the diagnoses of depression or cognitive impairment considered as a possibility. This focuses attention and should improve detection rates, resulting in an increase in referral of mild and early cases.

More than 50% of GPs do not use any tools to detect dementia or cognitive impairment (Audit Commission 2000), mainly because they are reluctant (O'Connor and Fertig 1993). The best start point is to *encourage the use of a short, simple instrument to detect cognitive impairment* that can be used easily in the surgery, perhaps within any single assessment procedure [e.g. the over-75 checks (Chew *et al.* 1994)] and can be incorporated into an agreed protocol with local services. Options that exist include:

- Mini-Mental State Examination (MMSE, Folstein *et al.* 1975): universal in dementia services, relatively easy to use, with minimal training, but with educational and language bias. It misses early cases and has no measure of executive function. It is considered long by GPs.
- Abbreviated Mental Test Score (AMTS, Hodkinson 1972): liked by many GPs who came through geriatric medicine. It is not a well-validated scale, which suffers even more as users often change it to suit. This gives wide variation in scores and interpretation.
- 7-minute screen (Solomon *et al.* 1997): useful test for early AD that uses four short tests to compile a score indicative of disease, but often takes more than the 7 minutes the title indicates. It involves using some materials, which puts GPs off. It may be better for surgery staff or CPNs when cognitive impairment is already demonstrated.
- 6-CIT (Katzman *et al.* 1983): an old test recently revalidated (Brooke and Bullock 1999) that uses six questions to determine cognitive impairment. These questions are weighted, and easily interpreted. It is available on the surgery computer (via EMIS) and is part of the Easy Care screening system that is being piloted across Europe as a

standardised dataset to follow up the elderly in the community, and so may become the preferred single assessment. GPs that have used the 6-CIT find it straightforward and quick.

Other tests include the Middlesex Elderly Assessment of Mental State (MEAMS, Golding 1989) and the Clifton Assessment Procedures for the Elderly (CAPE) (Pattie and Gilleard 1979), which have been favoured more by secondary services, and the DemTect (Kessler *et al.* 2000), which uses a combination of short tests to show the presence of quite mild cognitive impairment.

Whatever is the preferred test, it should be used as part of the referral across the service. All GPs should be encouraged to use it and set the cut-off scores for referral where there is mutual agreement to assess patients. This reduces fears that patients are being sent too early or inappropriately. What is needed is for the GP to feel they have confidently diagnosed cognitive impairment, anything more at this stage is a luxury. Using this system not only can low referring GPs be identified, but the mean level of cognitive impairment at which referrals take place can also be fed back to practices.

To develop this further, the short test could be accepted as the basis of a service referral from practice staff, district nurses, or, more adventurously, staff at NHS direct – making it unnecessary for everybody to see the GP first. Total access to the tests could be provided 24-hourly on a web site. The possibilities expand according to the resource available.

Any one of these tests could be used when the patient presents. None of them is diagnostic, and should not be used as such. We use the 6-CIT in Swindon, especially as it is part of the Easy Care single assessment in primary care that our local GPs have adopted. It is incorporated into the flow chart in Figure 3.3.

The other groups who need to help in aiding detection are the patients and carers. They often do not present with straightforward histories and hedge around the issue of memory loss due to fear of Alzheimer's disease. However, carers pick up signs of change early (Aneshensel and Pearlin 1995; Nolan and Cardock 1996). Public information to ease the interview with the GP and reduce the stigma of AD is needed – provided the specialist services are ready for the increased demand. Squeezing the GP between informed patients and unreactive services will help nobody.

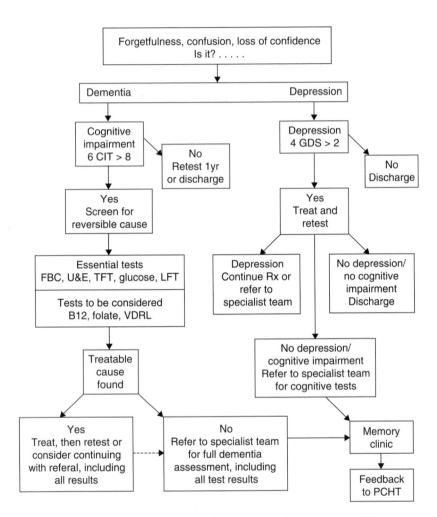

Figure 3.3 Integrated care pathway for dementia. Stage 1: recognising dementia

Summary

The main aims to assist detection in primary care are:

- to increase the number of early cases assessed
- to increase educational input to the surgeries – FMN recommendation 3 (Audit Commission 2000)
- to give a paradigm to increase awareness
- to decide on a simple yes/no instrument that can be used in the surgery to 'diagnose' the presence of cognitive impairment
- to consider offering it to other potential referrers
- to inform and educate patients and carers how to ask for help – FMN recommendations 1 and 2 (Audit Commission 2000).

Referral

Many myths hinder the process of referring early cases of dementia to specialists (Milne 1998). The first is that nothing can be done, so why bother (Audit Commission 2000). The second is that referring too many cases is a sign of weakness and counts against the GP. The third is a fear of making an inappropriate referral. The fourth is that there are so many cases out there, services would be snowed under.

Nothing can be done

This is clearly not the case as will be shown later, and *upbeat and enthusiastic services* engender a good relationship with GPs, especially if feedback from the referral is positive and speedy.

Too many referrals

Determining the aetiology and making a differential diagnosis in early dementia is a skilled process, and is important for treatment and prognostic purposes. In most circumstances it is a specialist practice. This means that detection is a role that should lead to referral, and that for dementia, failure to refer is a bigger problem than referring too much.

Fear of inappropriate referral

This can be overcome using a simple test.

Snowed under

Current services do not provide that well for early cases at present, and would be snowed under if all patients were suddenly referred. But in reality this would not be the case. What is needed is a gradual provision of more time for this patient group, particularly from the senior medical staff – indicating a change in their priorities. The commonest method to see this group is in *memory clinics*, the presence of which has been endorsed in the National Service Framework for older people (Department of Health 2001a). Setting up such services must now be a priority, as without them an increase in public knowledge and increasing referral rate will hit an unacceptable bottleneck and *waiting lists* will be unacceptably long. While it may not be a bad thing to have waiting lists – they do attract extra resource in the acute sector – it is better to plan strategically to try and avoid them. Many instruments and population datasets exist to aid this process (Isaacs and Neville 1975; Ely *et al.* 1996; Melzer *et al.* 1997; Melzer 1999) – but they may be an underestimate (Black *et al.* 1990). As services develop, there may be a delay in meeting demand – as the clinics are attempting to embrace a large unmet need. This delay needs to be agreed locally with the primary care group, and kept within recommended maximums if possible.

However, Table 3.1 does suggest that this will not be that easy in the UK, given the low numbers of specialists available. It is remarkable in many ways that comparative numbers of people actually do get seen here – either a testimony to hard work or overwork (or both).

The information requested by secondary care at referral should also be agreed. A short history and current medication are useful, but most

Table 3.1 Comparision of available specialists in UK, France and Germany

	UK	France	Germany
Neurologists	488	1300	7650[t]
Geriatricians	997	1000	580
Psychogeriatricians	545	6000*	4939[‡]

Clearly, the availability of expertise is uniquely low in the UK.
*Number of psychiatrists.
[t]2276 (+ 5374 special qualification related to neurology).
[‡]1851 (+ 3089 psychiatrists).

of this will be repeated in the initial assessment. Details of cardiovascular disorder and hypertensive history are important, as is proof of cognitive impairment. Some GPs will provide current basic blood tests to show they have looked for reversible causes (FBC, U&E, TFT, lipids and liver function). These need doing, though reversal of many of these causes does not seem to help the cognitive loss. Part of the protocol locally can agree who will do what. It is better in many ways if other possible treatable conditions have been identified before the first appointment. Figure 3.3 summarises the processes of detection and referral in the form of a flow chart.

Summary

Mechanisms to improve referral from primary care are:

- to be upbeat and enthusiastic about what services can offer – and give good feedback
- to show that understanding the aetiology and differential diagnosis in early cases needs specialist skills
- to make referral the norm, with no filters other than using the simple cognitive test selected
- to agree a referral protocol that is short and easy to use, including agreement as to who does initial blood tests
- to provide memory clinics or similar services
- to use waiting lists constructively and agree delays with local primary caregiver.

4 ASSESSMENT PROCESSES

Referrals need to be clearly processed and moved in to an efficient assessment system. This really needs to be shared by health and social services in an integrated way. Many services now enjoy a much healthier relationship with local social services, but proper integration is rarer, and since the Health Act (Department of Health 1999), the formation of care trusts has not been rapid. Some debate whether a single assessment is achievable (Philp 1997), while others have published models (e.g. EPICS; Hunter and Wistow 1990). However, structural change does not need to occur prior to good joint working. The following ten points are good indicators of an integrated approach, and many can be negotiated with the services as they are configured now:

- consistent initial screening process irrespective of who took the original referral
- assessment of need accepted for Care Programme Approach (CPA) and care management
- single care plans
- single care manager across all agencies
- inter-agency management
- policy on confidentiality and sharing across agencies
- common complaints procedure
- shared information systems
- joint communication strategies to keep users/carers informed
- CPA coordinator to start process working – probably less needed in mature services.

It makes sense if all referrals are handled in a similar fashion and that information flow is as easy as possible. Factors that assist in creating an environment that assists such flow include:

- shared bases for health and social services
- all referrals, for both health and social services, going to a single point of entry

- allocation to all areas of the service at a single meeting
- health and social services using combined, commonly accepted paperwork
- agreed definitions of unmet need
- CPA and care management being treated as one entity
- free access to information for all staff who need it.

If all of the above can be arranged, the move from referral to assessment should occur seamlessly and the right person be allocated to make the first visit.

Evaluating the patient

The assessment of dementia has been described in numerous consensuses, and evidence-based documents (Waldemar *et al.* 2000; Knopman *et al.* 2001). In summary, to arrive at a differential diagnosis, the following steps need to be taken:

- general history taking
- neurological examination
- cognitive testing, plus assessment of function and behaviour
- referral for ancillary testing, e.g. neuropsychology, imaging, laboratory tests and occasionally EEG or lumbar puncture
- identification and treatment of vascular factors in dementia
- diagnosis and treatment of seizures and extrapyramidal disturbances
- diagnosis, or differential diagnosis, and aetiology (where possible) evaluated
- advice to patient, carer and referring physician on all aspects of diagnosis and treatment.

How these investigations are done and what is included or left out depends on a number of factors (van Crevel *et al.* 1999), usually around availability of resources, for example, neuropsychology. Traditionally we look for reversible causes, even though not many seem to reverse in practice (Clarfield 1988). Whilst a one-shop stop is attractive, delays in imaging usually makes this an impossible dream, and waiting lists for scans add to the difficulties. Although scans may now be an important part of the assessment (Foster *et al.* 1999), it would be imprudent to order them in advance of appointments, as far too many would then be done. As a result, assessment tends to be a two-stage process.

Stage 1

- History, examination, neuropsychology, bloods, ECG
- Assessment of function, behaviour and carer burden
- Stage dementia and provisional diagnosis
- Order imaging and any other investigations, e.g. EEG

Stage 2

- Look at results of all tests
- Make diagnosis and discuss with patient and carer
- Talk of options and set expectations
- Set up treatment plan and record baselines
- Offer post-diagnostic counselling, if required or available.

Ideally these visits will be around 6 weeks apart, but the time to get tests done will set the period. Where the assessment is done does not matter particularly. Traditionally they have been performed in people's homes but memory clinics are becoming more mainstream – especially with mild-to-moderate dementia, where patients are less unwell, *the domiciliary visit (DV) gives less information* and the patient is more amenable to a clinic-based approach.

As a result, the memory clinic becomes a sensible entity, which is usually hospital based and consultant led. The system can be designed to collect most of the information in a sensible order, maximising the use of everybody's time. This allows the patient to receive a full assessment and diagnosis at a pace that suits them (some tests can still be performed at home), and presents the diagnosing doctor with the information they require. Giving the diagnosis has been a subject of debate (Rice and Warner 1994; Maguire *et al.* 1996), but it is generally felt that people should be told (Fearnley and McLennan 1997; Pinner 2000), especially with the use of medication (Meyers 1997). Post-diagnostic psychological work is now an expanding area of interest.

This is a very medical, almost neurological model – but that is what occurs in dementia services around the rest of the world where neurology and geriatrics provide the bulk of the care. In the UK, though, the clinic has the advantage of being embedded in a larger community model that offers more choices and holistic care. Medical clinics in old age psychiatry services therefore represent a progressive recognition of the psychiatrist's medical skills, offering an environment where doctors can exert their two main contributions: diagnosis and treatment.

The role of the consultant in modern services

The modern dementia service is starting to look very different and the focus of the consultant will change with it. Old age psychiatry has become a huge field with areas ranging from complex psychopharmacology through community outreach services into palliative care. I believe that the field is now so big that sub-specialisation is becoming inevitable. This may not necessarily mean having whole jobs sub-specialised, but I think to offer a balanced service, the local areas need to agree special interests for the senior clinicians, so that important parts of the field are covered appropriately.

The days of the small consultant fiefdoms, where the consultant does everything, are numbered. It makes little sense, and although many consultants have leadership skills, not all have. The drive for lower catchment areas and increased numbers has worked, though sometimes at the expense of other community services. This now means that groups of consultants can aggregate and look at what is needed in the area, and match skills and interests to need. Thus, an area may have a consultant who is very keen on memory clinic work and another who likes the community assessments more, and another who prefers in-patient work. Rather than do all three on an arbitrary geographical basis, it may be more sensible to arrange work according to interest, ensuring that patients always get the most enthusiastic staff. We are a stable and mature group who should be able to achieve this arrangement – even perhaps across Trust boundaries. There is certainly no place now for an organisation to have a lone old age psychiatrist performing all roles, and this should be actively discouraged. It also makes arranging on-call rotas for the speciality an easier task, as having pooled rotas with general psychiatry is no longer sensible given the widening disparity between the fields; that, on clinical governance grounds alone, is exposing patients of both groups to unnecessary risks.

Thus, consultants will now have increased flexibility in their choice of job plan. By practising what they are interested in, they are more likely to perform or utilise research and modern methodology. Trainees will benefit from this, and in turn choose their clinical sessions from a menu of special interests rather than aligned to just one consultant. This broadens their experience and makes them even more obviously super-numerary, as their alignment to just one team will be less. This allows the educational supervision to take place outside the straight hierarchy models, and hopefully produce more rounded specialists at the comple-tion of training.

This model strengthens and makes clearer the consultant's role. It may mean that traditional methods need re-evaluation, and for many this may be anathema – especially the decline in domiciliary visits. Of dementia work today, 75% appears to be based on older models, but Oscar Wilde did say that 'just because everybody agrees on something, does not mean that it is not still completely preposterous', and contin-uing as we are may well be the case here.

What constitutes a memory clinic?

The term memory clinic arose in the USA in the late 1970s. It was origi-nally associated with research rather than mainstream practice and up to 1995 there were only 25 or so in the UK (Wright and Lindesay 1995). After 1997, and the launch of donepezil, many memory clinics have sprung up across the UK, so now there are 120 at least, and the mention of their desirability in the national service framework promises more.

However, they are a mixed group of clinic types, some being almost virtual. The different types include:

- full blown assessment of all memory disorders of all age, including neuropsychology, imaging and genetics. These are often research clinics with close links to clinical trials
- dementia clinics with full assessments as above, and prescribing of cholinesterase inhibitors
- dementia clinics with simple measurements and prescribing
- prescribing clinics/services set up to get the cholinesterase inhibitors to the patients
- complex home assessment and treatment.

What the clinic offers will depend on the available resources, including the interests of the consultant staff. The comprehensive memory services are more expensive and the need for imaging in many cases means a new expense, often not currently budgeted for. The commonest clinics are the small dementia clinics whose main role is prescribing. Several issues arise when planning the memory clinic provision in a service, as follows.

- What are the services around at present? How many clinics are nearby – do I need a new one or shall I work in another? Overcoming the tendency of the consultant to want to do and be in charge of everything is always a test.
- What is the most appropriate clinic here? For example, if I want an all-singing, all-dancing clinic, is it likely to happen, especially as this is a rural patch and the wait for imaging is 8 months.
- What infrastructure already exists in the service? What is going on already that I can group together to support the development of the clinic and get some way towards my aim?
- How will the NICE money be allocated? The money health authorities calculate to implement NICE guidance is not exhaustive. The aim really should be to prescribe to as many patients as possible, so any spend on infrastructure should be kept to a minimum. If not, it would seem that money for treating patients may get diverted into setting up services that should arguably be funded in other ways.
- What does the clinic need to do? Do I want to do complex assessment of memory disorder, so expanding my patient group, or do I want a treatment centre for dementia. Whatever, there is sense in splitting assessment and prescribing into separate clinics. This should improve the way patients are processed and audit information is collected. It also separates those receiving treatment from those who are not, which has certain advantages.

If prescribing is a separate process, then in a single area consultants can choose whether to work in a central memory assessment centre and/or the local prescribing service. In this way any consultant can design and work in a system that suits their style of working and their interests, for if memory assessment is not their main interest, they can choose to use the central assessment service, while retaining the prescribing relationship with their own area patients.

Can we standardise the clinics? Memory clinics are springing up on an *ad hoc* basis, doing broadly the same work using a variety of tests. Some do a lot of imaging, others very little. Neuropsychological testing can take 10 minutes to 2 hours. It would be useful to have some standardisation across clinics to better understand how best to use them and their impact. To this end, a UK Memory Clinic Association is now developing a minimum dataset, and looking at using computerised assessments in the routine clinic.

Commissioning memory clinics

To do this successfully needs to have all the questions above developed into a business case, and then costed. Table 4.1 gives some approximate costings of the components of a standard assessment clinic, and does not include any drug costs. This suggests that each session will cost about £20 000 per annum, in assessing 100 new patients and 150 follow-ups. Some of these costs can be reduced by the choice of clinic type, and some will be catered for already. It is important when designing any new service to be aware of what agreements are already established, for example, volume of blood tests at the local acute unit, or who may be seeing these patients currently. A sudden increase in demand will need a resource to meet it, and existing resource for the service should be transferred where possible.

New services attract referrals, so commissioning should reflect the projected numbers that will be seen and waiting times need agreeing. Having a waiting list is inevitable, as seen elsewhere in the NHS. However, if the aim of the service is to shift to early dementia, then one clinic will not be enough, and part of the commissioning will need to be an estimate of the expected total demand using well defined models (Melzer *et al.*

Table 4.1 Typical costings for one memory clinic session

		Cost (£)
Consultant time	1 session	130
Psychology assistant	1 session	20
Nurse	1 session	40
Lab work	2 new, 3 follow-up	15
CT/MRI		40/140 per item
Neuropsychology input		30
Overheads/admin		100
	Total	415* per clinic

£21 500 per year, per clinic session.
*Incorporates average across the range of CT and MRI quoted costs

1997). This needs to be aligned to how the service as a whole will create further clinics to meet demand, probably by stopping doing something else, particularly the doctors. This move towards such a clinic base will need to be explained and agreed with colleagues locally.

Patients presenting *later* in the illness still need many of the assessments detailed above, but *extra information will be gathered by performing the examination in the community setting*. The patients are often not so well and making them travel to a hospital is often a hindrance to them and unnecessary. Consequently, the memory clinic should concentrate on patients above a defined cut-off, while below this, the traditional home-based services continue. Again, standardised assessments are easier to communicate, and much of the information at home can be gathered in advance of any necessary doctor's visit. With earlier treatment, hopefully this patient group will diminish in size, and the needs will change – reduction in this activity can be factored into the business plans as a long-term release of resource.

The role of the Community Mental Health Team (CMHT) in modern services

The CMHT is the *fundamental part of the community services*, and offers a variety of assessment and care options that hopefully can address most of the patients' and carers' needs, especially where health and social services have managed to integrate. *Using the community team to assess the more advanced patients* at home is highly appropriate for several reasons:

- most of the patients' needs will be met by the non-medical specialities;
- the model provides the flexibility to meet the needs of those with dementia who live alone (Social Services Inspectorate 1997) and have different requirements (Alzheimer's Disease Society 1994);
- delay may be built into a system that relies on a consultant visit as there is inevitably fewer of them than anyone else;
- it is recommended in FMN 4 and 5 (Audit Commission 2000);
- the domiciliary system is expensive, and often used to get an appointment with the consultant for the least appropriate patients. When consultants syphon off these patients, they compromise the relationship they have as part of the CMHT.

Unfortunately, several barriers have historically got in the way of the formation of these teams:

- The traditional *dominance of medicine and nursing* has meant many so-called multidisciplinary teams are bidiscipline only, sometimes with fractions of other disciplines, if lucky.
- *Leadership* has always been an issue, with the consultant often assuming the leadership role even when this may not be the most sensible option – a problem perpetuated by calling the CMHT 'Dr X's team', and the college liking teams to be broken neatly into consultant-sized patches.
- There is often lack of understanding of what the other disciplines actually offer.
- Most disciplines insist that only senior practitioners can work in the community, which means that all the nurses are G grades and the first appointment of a new discipline is often very expensive.
- The Royal College of Psychiatrists has pushed very hard to achieve *low catchment area sizes for consultants*. Consultants are costly and often appointed at the expense of developing community teams. A strategy to develop both is required at the outset.
- Historically every discipline has collected and kept its own information.
- Health and Social Services have varied levels of cooperation.
- The processes of care management and the care programme approach have kept this divide open, as they come to represent the different cultures.
- *Confidentiality* has always been a barrier to holistic care.

Putting together a CMHT

Much is spoken of the CMHT but it is usually not that multidisciplinary in nature, and even when it is, not that much of a team – that is, an integrated organic being that learns and develops as one. A collection of individuals in the same room is not a team. To become so needs shared ideals and a common understanding of the aims, and how each member contributes.

To get to this level of operation takes some time and so must be planned. This involves several steps, as follows.

24

Identify all resources and pool them

Before deciding what you need it is best to see what you have – across all providing agencies.

Look at grades

Traditionally, high grades work in the community. Lower grades can do a lot of the work under supervision, and agreeing new job specifications with the professional heads is an important early step. From here the structure for professional supervision and appraisal will take shape – ensuring quality and personal development.

Look at skill mix – professional and personal

A person with dementia has various needs (Figure 4.1), as does the carer. In order to meet these needs, the team has to offer staff with varying skills. Nursing is commonly present, but occupational therapists (OTs) to assess function are rarer, with physiotherapists to help disabilities, and speech and language therapists to assist with communication problems found much less frequently. There are a variety of disciplines possible and it is important to derive a balance of these skills as appropriate to the area. The Community Psychiatric Nurses (CPNs) cannot and should not do it all.

When developing the skill mix it is important to do so collectively. There was once a fear of creating a communal all-skilled worker to suit all needs. Whilst perhaps attractive to policy makers, it would have been a disaster in practice. Gathering all the disciplines together in a

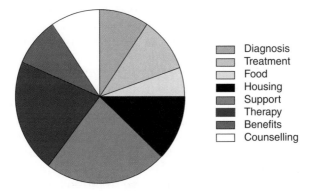

Figure 4.1   The needs of a person with dementia

room and telling each other what they do is an interesting experience. Three things should emerge:

- About 70% of what we all do is the same, so documenting this and using it to create the basis of a common assessment makes a good deal of sense. This does not create a common worker, but does avoid duplication, and will help stop a series of workers asking the same questions, creating the impression for the patients and carers that we never speak to each other (sometimes perhaps rightly).
- All team members understand what their colleagues actually do. This is surprisingly not always the case. The development process improves communication and helps match patient needs to the correct person.
- The specialist nature of each discipline's work is highlighted and in fact initial fears of homogenisation are replaced with a true sense of specialism.

Personal skills are often forgotten. Staff skilled in issues such as bereavement, cognitive therapy or counselling, irrespective of their professional skill, will be missed if these extra skills are not replaced when they leave. Knowing the complete skills set is an important task for the community team manager. Good services may extend this model beyond their own sphere – encompassing home care and other sectors as well (FMN recommendation 6; Audit Commission 2000).

Develop common values
The team needs to understand, own, and know why it is there and what its boundaries are. Without this, the development of a common understanding will be difficult, and the next step almost impossible.

Design common instruments and processes
If the team is going to function as one, it needs to act as one. Common assessment tools and paperwork help this happen and make communication more effective and seamless. The crucial boundary is the health and social services one where acceptance of a common tool speeds up services to the person at home (FMN recommendation 14; Audit Commission 2000).

To do this effectively does involve some suspension of old boundaries. Figure 4.2 gives an example of the care programme form used in Swindon,

Department of Old Age Psychiatry
Avon and Wiltshire Mental Health Partnership NHS Trust

CARE PROGRAMME APPROACH MEETING   **CONFIDENTIAL**

Record of Initial / Review (No ___) / Discharge meeting on ___/___/_____

Surname	Forenames	D.O.B	Hospital No / Patient Identifier

Address:		Sex:	Marital Status:
			☐ M
		☐ M	☐ W
			☐ S
Tel:		☐ F	☐ D
			☐ Co-habit

Consultant:	GP:	Address:
	Tel:	

Invited to CPA meeting:	Role:	Attended (please tick)

Interpreter Required: Yes ☐ No ☐	Advocate arranged: Yes ☐ No ☐

Type of CPA: (please tick as appropriate)	Minimal ☐	Complex ☐

Risk Assessment carried out? Yes ☐ No ☐	On Supervision Register? Yes ☐ No ☐

☐   Subject to statutory supervision by probation service
☐   Subject to section 25
☐   Subject to guardianship
☐   Subject to conditional discharge Section 37/41
☐   Subject to Section 117 (i.e. currently detained on Section 3 or 37)
☐   Subject to Criminal Procedure (Insanity and Unfitness to Plead Act 1991)
☐   Subject to a Section of the Mental Health Act (Please Specify):

Evaluation of Current Care Plan / Significant changes since last meeting:

Keyworker:	Care Manager: (If different)
Location:	Location:
Tel No:	Tel No:

In an Emergency:
9.00am – 7.30pm   Please contact your Keyworker
Weekdays   OR the Duty Officer on 07000 782 653

Out of Hours and Weekends   Please contact the Emergency Duty Service on 01793 465 333

Review Due:	Month	Year

Figure 4.2   The care programme forms used in Swindon

27

NEEDS ASSESSMENT				
1. Daily Living Activity	Yes ☐ No ☐	6. Emotional Wellbeing	Yes ☐ No ☐
2. Household Management	Yes ☐ No ☐	7. Social Relationships	Yes ☐ No ☐
3. Access Mobility	Yes ☐ No ☐	8. Communication	Yes ☐ No ☐
4. Accommodation	Yes ☐ No ☐	9. Day Time Occupation	Yes ☐ No ☐
5. General Health	Yes ☐ No ☐	10. Finance / Benefit Check	Yes ☐ No ☐

NEEDS IDENTIFIED

RISKS IDENTIFIED

1. Deliberate Self Harm	Yes ☐ No ☐	3. Abuse	Yes ☐ No ☐
2. Neglect	Yes ☐ No ☐	4. Aggression / Other	Yes ☐ No ☐

Where risk identified – assessment and management plan attached

CHANGES IN NEED / RISKS

CARER STRESS:

None ☐   Mild ☐   Moderate ☐   Severe ☐

Has the carer requested an assessment?   Yes ☐ No ☐

Figure 4.2 *Continued*

28

CARE PLAN (including any changes)	Action / By Date:

RESOURCE SHORTFALL

Action Taken:-   Shortfall reporting, Form Date:

Significant indicators which may suggest Relapse / Breakdown of Care Plan:	Action to be taken:	By Whom:
Proposed Hospital Discharge / extended leaving date:	Proposed discharge address if different from home address:	

If appropriate, reasons for User / Carer not attending CPA meeting / not signing CPA.

User's nominated contact (i.e. Carer / Friend)	
Name:	Address:
Tel:	
Signed:......................................(User) / Carer	Date:..
Signed:......................................(Keyworker)	Date:..
Responsible Medical Officer:..	Date:..
Social Services:..	Date:..

CIRCULATION: User / Carer / Keyworker / Ward Area / GP / Other

Figure 4.2 *Continued*

Date Commencing:

FOR DAILY / WEEKLY CARE

Service Provider (Including informal carer)	Monday	Tuesday	Wednesday	Thursday	Friday	Saturday	Sunday	Comments / Start Date
Service Name Tel:								
Service Name Tel:								
Service Name Tel:								
Service Name Tel:								
Service Name: Tel:								

NAME: ADDRESS:

Figure 4.2 *Continued*

following completion of a common assessment tool. The initial assessment does not need to be completed in its entirety at the first visit, but some information is crucial in order to access services, until the final care programme is prepared. This means that in integrated services, social workers will be doing some assessment of cognition and nurses gathering some basic financial information – with all team members giving out financial advice and direction. This may offend some traditional sensitivities, but does ensure the patient gets immediate access to services after one visit, rather than wait on several lists for all the information to be gathered. Putting the patient first highlights the absurdity of some of our systems – and in some cases exposes them as even discriminatory.

Agree a risk assessment and management policy

With large numbers of patients being managed by a team of staff, it is important to have a risk assessment screen to ensure that those who are, or who are becoming, at risk can be consistently picked up. Many tools exist but few are specific for the needs of the elderly. An example of an elderly specific one is shown in Table 4.2. This was developed by one of our CPNs, and has worked consistently well in our department, targeting the high scorers for a proper assessment and focusing resource appropriately. Identifying risk is important, accepting that people are allowed to take risks and helping minimise them is a key role for the service – eliminating risk is less often the objective.

Allow learning time in everybody's working week

Most disciplines do not get the time off each week that doctors in training achieve as a right. A modern service will build such time into its strategic planning, so that all staff get at least a half day for personal development. This may compromise a heavy workload, but doing more at the expense of this development time leads to unhealthy and restless staff. The best way to improve services is to have many staff in further training, with their development matched to their own and the department's needs. If projects are then about the team's work, the team will be kept current and innovation will be captured. An example of that is the risk assessment described above, created for a degree dissertation. Making space for staff to develop is crucial if a learning environment is what is truly required. The rewards are better services, higher retention, easier recruitment and often, the time staff take out from work is supported financially by the educational consortia.

Table 4.2 Older people service risk assessment form, initial review

Patient name   DOB   Date   Case no.

Deliberate self-harm	Score	Neglect	Score	Abuse	Score	Aggression (to others)	Score
Previous serious attempt	12	Fires or evidence of burns (carpet, furniture, clothes, self, etc.)	10	**Carer factors**		Content of delusions indicates harm to specific others	14
Formulated plan	10	Inadequate fluid intake	10	Poor premorbid relationship	10	Past forensic history	10
Alcohol abuse	9	Appliances left unattended, e.g. gas on but not lit, etc.	10	Claim of abuse (patient to carer)	10	**Related to dementia**	
Depressive illness (current)	6	Inadequate or inappropriate food, or lack of access to food	10	Previous psychiatric history	6	Paranoid delusions	10
Apparently minor attempt (a few tablets)	5	Exploitation, e.g. money stolen, door left open	6	Current depression	6	Resisting intervention	10
Severe physical illness	5	Wandering, e.g. into road, returned by police or neighbours	6	Alcohol or drug abuse	6	Hitting others	10
Long duration of mental illness or previous MHA	5	Poor compliance with medication	5	Financial properties or dependency	5	Shouting/swearing at others	7
Severe uncontrolled pain	5	Lack of adequate heating	5	**Patient factors**		Sexually disinhibited	7

Expression of hopelessness	4	Poor quality food, e.g. left out of fridge, rotting or past sell-by date	5	Claim of abuse (carer to patient)	10	Delirium	7
Recent significant bereavement	3	Deterioration in personal hygiene, e.g. smell of urine/faeces on clothes, wearing same clothes	4	Aggression towards carer	6		/75
Severe insomnia	3	Deterioration in standards of house maintenance and cleanliness, resulting in a dangerous environment	4	Marked decline in cognition (rapid or recent)	6	**Falls**	
Living alone	3			Unusual bruising	6	History of falls	15
Unable to assess mental state, e.g. mute	3			Repetitive antisocial behaviour	4	MMSE <24	15
Poor rapport with the patient	1			Carer assessment	Y/N	Polypharmacy	15
Male	1			Need for carer assessment	Y/N	Cardiological/neurological problems	15
Overall total	/75	Overall total	/75	Overall total	/75	Visual problems	15
						Overall total	/75

In any section, <15 = low risk, monitor; 16–30 = medium risk, review; >31 = high risk, immediate action.

Signed...

Hold regular time out away from work

Taking time to discuss and develop the above processes is crucial. There should be regular weekly meetings set aside for the business of the team, which is conducted separately from the clinical supervision of patients in the community. This meeting is most effective with a structured agenda (see Table 4.3) and a rotating chair. There is a macho position adopted in the NHS where taking this time out of a week is not real work and it stops patients being seen. This is not usually the case, and is a practical way of achieving an old aphorism of 'working smarter, not harder'.

The other time away from work should be in the form of regular away days – at least yearly and probably 6-monthly. Here, assessment of where things are can be matched to the vision of the team and action planning can keep the strategic direction.

Table 4.3 Structured agenda for team meetings

Minutes of previous meeting
Matters arising
Developments
Courses
  • feedback from
  • courses to attend
Information sharing
Team/any other business
New case allocation
Clinical feedback

Replace staff according to need

The old days of every discipline tightly guarding its own budget must stop. A mature team will treat someone leaving as an opportunity to discuss what they currently need most to assist their work. Thus, if a CPN leaves, the priority may be for a new occupational therapist (OT), and if this is the common agreement, the system needs to be flexible enough to do this. This is most easily achieved by having all budgets with the community team manager, and service level agreements with the discipline heads to prevent sudden unilateral decisions.

34

Arrange the care management process

Patients accepted into the dementia services will be placed in a care management process (FMN recommendation 13; Audit Commission 2000). At present, different terms have represented different agencies and different names have been given to key players. This has proved confusing to patients, carers and staff alike. Care management is traditionally a social services term and is a form of resource management. Care programme approach (CPA) is a health process, often relegated to an audit phenomenon by which the paper trail is used to show that services are meeting basic requirements. Care planning is our job. I would contend these are all the same – especially in the new care trusts, where community resources are now becoming pooled. Projects to look at pooled resources are needed now, to complement those that have been done on a single agency basis (Stewart *et al.* 1999).

Unless this historic standoff is resolved, patients will continue to get a poorer service, and the only people who will prosper are those who still offer training days on the integration of CPA and care management – now with a new acronym ICPA (integrated care programme approach). Names are less relevant than robust and transparent processes.

Our service has a care management process, where there is a core team of care managers (called so simply because it describes what they do) – derived from nursing and social work. The care managers are senior grades supported by lower grades and support workers. The care manager is the named person for the patient or carer to contact and has the responsibility to coordinate all activity around them, including that of the responsible medical officer (RMO). They relate with the team and the primary care team, and maintain the seamlessness as far as possible. They also keep this care management role when patients are admitted, either into the service beds, or the acute unit – where they often see patients first as they have most of the relevant information. Care managers also arrange admissions, prioritising them amongst themselves (only using the consultant where a difficult decision is needed) and set up all respite. The care manager is the main agent of continuity, shared care protocols and review - as relevant as, if not more relevant than, the medical staff involved.

Another care management issue is which staff should do it. Small teams try and use everybody, but whilst this shares load, it does pose other dilemmas. Using the small amount of time available from therapists to perform care management is not a good use of their time, as they often need to come in for a quick assessment or make an intervention and withdraw – engaging in long-term assessment is not usually needed unless circumstances dictate. It is probably best not to use them for care management, nor the doctors, whose day-to-day availability is variable and their main function is not to arrange care.

The best way to picture this is that the care manager opens a folder (as on a computer) for a patient and at any one time other members of staff may contribute a file to that folder. For example, an OT may do a bathing assessment and a psychologist may do some work with the carer.

Outer core: Specialised input
Inner core: Care management

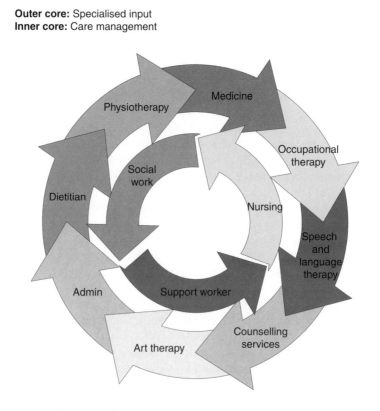

Figure 4.3 Structure of an integrated CMHT – inner care management and outer specialised input

Neither has to formally open a new case (folder) as they can document what they are doing in combined files within the existing folder. This avoids duplication, and stops patients appearing on too many caseloads, thereby distorting service figures. This model is best represented by a two-ring scenario (Figure 4.3) with a central care management function and an outer group of available specialisms to call on.

This system works well internally, but can also clarify roles externally. It is easy to explain, and if giving supplementary advice to other teams, the principles remain the same. Offering a simple assessment to a geriatric colleague in a one-off assessment is acting as a file in their particular folder. The only slight difference is when a care manager gets involved in an ongoing manner with another external folder, for example, a non-EMI social services case. Here their contribution is not as the care manager, but as the key worker from our department.

Agree relationship with primary care

General practice assumes 24-hour responsibility for patients and is often a point of call for patients with dementia. CPA also means a 24-hour commitment as well, so shared care agreements need to be explicitly made. The care manager needs to relate to the practice, and monthly contact about the patients they manage is useful. There are various models of working together, ranging from all but physical care being provided from the secondary service, to the GP doing most of the care and using the CMHT as required. It is often felt by GPs that they should have their own CPN. This may be achievable in some centres, but is probably slightly retrograde as splitting nursing from the care management process breaks up the team, reduces the supervision and deprives nurses of true multidisciplinary interaction. Usually GPs ask for nurses because they feel they improve communication – other strategies will deal with this better. Some still think nurses will do counselling, for which most are not qualified; but this is less often the case.

In years to come the CMHT's work may become mainstream primary care, especially as all elderly services will logically end up in the PCT. At present, the developing dementia services need to grow and learn where they can best achieve maximum potential.

Provide appropriate supervision and management

The CMHT is providing the bulk of the community work across a broad range of disciplines and scenarios. The care managers need appropriate supervision, which may be from different disciplines. This needs to be defined and regulated and any problems about the supervisor dealt with. The management of the work of the team is via its manager, professional supervision is via professional leads. If this is accepted, structures fall in to place.

One aspect of the supervision is to furnish staff with some basic tools to help judge situations.

'Why me' and 'why now' are the first two questions to be answered in the response situation. If neither has a clear answer, the case needs discussion with another team member in order to make sure that action at this time is appropriate. Going in at the wrong time can lead to long-term difficulties that a little preplanning can avoid.

'What's the problem' also needs clearly identifying, as often with more advanced patients with dementia it is someone else's problem that is being dealt with, sometimes inappropriately.

Utilising these tools can train patients, carers and referrers how best to use the service to meet their needs. Over time this creates a better working relationship and reduces the amount of firefighting that gets done. This reduces the rate of emergency situations.

Dilemmas in the modernisation of assessment process

Modernising the assessment process does throw up some interesting dilemmas, as to do it logically and effectively serves to challenge some fundamental principles.

- It creates two streams in the process, that start at the common referral entry point:
- the more medical memory assessment process of the early to early moderate stage dementias, which requires diversion of specialist time, and budgets for investigation and imaging; the improving CMHT assessment of the moderate-to-severe dementias.
- By having one entry point to the service, the more medical referrals are allocated by the team to the clinic/diagnostic service. This ends any doctor-to-doctor communication that bypasses the CMHT, making the access to the team easier and rendering the traditional DV obsolete.
- The early-stage patients usually come under the care of the memory clinic, and do not require the CMHT until a little later. This is a

service that does not fulfil a direct function for the CMHT, as all others have in the past. So new relationship issues need addressing, to avoid the CMHT being involved too late. Using *trigger questions* in the clinic (for example, checking that the carer is still well and coping, or whether the patient's level of functional dependency has deteriorated) can start a referral process to the team to ensure this does not occur.

• It calls into question which part of the illness is best suited for GP supervision. This will be developed more in the review section.

• It reverses the current scenario where specialist assessment begins with moderate dementia, making the need for understanding and using early detection and assessment tools paramount.

Health economic assessments in dementia

Dementia consumes a lot of resource, about £5 billion a year of state funding in the UK (Bosanquet *et al.* 1998; Souetre *et al.* 1999) – which would be £14 billion if carer time was also costed (Max *et al.* 1995). It is known that resource use and caregiver burden increase with the severity of the illness (Gray and Fenn 1993) and this predicts institutionalisation. Community services, while providing better person-centred care, are no less expensive (Livingston *et al.* 1997). It is also known that at this stage quality of life for the patient and carer are diminishing.

To assess the impact of our interventions, we often look at patient- and carer-centred variables to estimate change in disease state or improvement in perceived quality of life. But the other side of the coin needed to show the value of our intervention is reduction in resource utilisation. Such measures include:

• number of visits to GP, hospital and social services by patient and carer;
• support services at home, e.g. home care, meals-on-wheels, etc.;
• caregiver time: supervision and assistance;
• institutionalisation.

It is therefore odd that data concerning resource utilisation is not routinely collected, and this omission should be rectified in a modern service. Simple data like date of presentation to the service, date of onset of symptoms, time of institutionalisation, and date of death offer good indicators of service effect. Caregiver diaries and logs of services provided show resources used. This information is crucial for planning and can indicate real-time effects (Kavanagh *et al.* 1993). We have not concentrated enough on monetary measures, which is part of what contributes to our current resource shortfall. We do not have clear ideas of what we need, but, perhaps worse is that any savings we may have created elsewhere in our care system to date may not be directly attributed, and consequently lost rather than reinvested.

To date, most economic work has been based on modelling, usually from clinical trial data (Ernst *et al.* 1997; Stern *et al.* 1997; Stewart *et al.* 1998) or attempts to calculate health utilities (Neumann *et al.* 1999). Real data is needed to answer the necessary questions.

Health economic modelling: the AHEAD model

J. Jaime Caro, Alex Ward and Judith O'Brien

The Assessing Health Economics in Alzheimer's Disease (AHEAD) model, a joint initiative between Janssen-Cilag and Shire Pharmaceuticals, was developed to address the long-term health and economic impact of managing patients with Alzheimer's disease. AHEAD predicts when a patient will require full-time care (FTC). The need for FTC is a function of the dependency that results from declining cognitive and functional ability as well as the appearance of behavioural problems and other factors.

Patients who do not yet require FTC are assumed to live either at home or in a residence that does not provide extensive nursing care. Patients who have deteriorated to the point where FTC is required may reside in an institution such as a nursing home or may be cared for in less intensive settings or even at home. The requirements for care are modelled over time, and the relevant costs are attributed accordingly.

The model forecasts outcomes for patients over the course of up to 10 years using equations that use an index score that incorporates multiple patient characteristics to estimate the risks of requiring FTC and of death as a function of time. Full details of the model and the predictive equations have been published elsewhere (Caro *et al.* 2001). For FTC predictions, the index includes the presence of extrapyramidal symptoms (EPS), the presence of psychotic symptoms, age at onset of cognitive symptoms, duration of illness, and cognitive score. Death predictions were based on an index that consists of EPS, duration of illness, gender and cognitive score.

Cost inputs for the model have been developed based on estimates of the health-care resources used in the UK (Kavanagh *et al.* 1995; Staton 1996; Bosanquet *et al.* 1998; Souetre *et al.* 1999) and expressed in 2001 British pounds (Netten *et al.* 1998; Scottish Health Service 2000). The monthly cost for nursing home care was estimated at £2250, and for FTC in the community to be £300. The services included in these cost estimates are the cost of formal (paid) care: hospital stays, visits to health-care professionals (physician, or nurse), nursing home care, and other paid services used (Meals on Wheels, day care, hours of home care). Some of the services included are not always reimbursed and, thus, are often paid for by the family. This broadens the perspective of these analyses beyond that of a comprehensive payer for medical care.

The model can be used to estimate the cumulative costs and outcomes of patients with various characteristics. For example, in one analysis, patient characteristics from two clinical trials were used as the inputs into the predictive equations, and forecasts were made for up to 10 years (Netten 1998; Getsios *et al.* 2001). When these patients were modelled without receiving treatment with a cholinesterase inhibitor, 40% of patients remaining alive were predicted to require FTC within 3 years, and 60% within 5 years. The resulting costs of caring for each patient were estimated to be, on average, £26 200 over 5 years and institutional care accounted for 62% of this cost. Even within 3 years, approximately half of the costs were estimated to be due to institutional care.

The impact of changes in the delivery of health-care services – for example, in order to reduce the proportion of patients receiving FTC in an institution – can be estimated using this model. For example, if the use of institutional care was reduced from the estimated 59% used by the model currently to 49%, then the average cumulative costs within 3 years are reduced by 7.5%. Thus, for every 100 patients with mild-to-moderate Alzheimer's disease who do not need FTC today, this change in delivery of care would be expected to save £118 000 over the next 3 years. Over an additional 2 years, the costs would drop by 9% and the savings would increase to £240 000.

This model has also been used to estimate the potential economic impact of treating patients with Alzheimer's disease based on the shorter-term data collected in clinical trials. For example, one recent analysis examined treatment with the new cholinesterase inhibitor, galantamine. This study indicated that the predicted health benefits from galantamine in terms of delaying the time to FTC are likely substantial enough to offset the treatment costs and reduce the overall cost of managing Alzheimer's disease in Canada.

Carers

Carers need informal and formal assessments throughout the stages of the disease (Twigg 1992; Levin 1997). These should be in line with the national Carers Charter. Local services need to furnish information about prognosis, possible breaks from caring and alternative ways of caring, along with acknowledgement of the work being done – and how it increases with severity.

Carers are an important resource, as they have first-hand experience of the disease. They come up with ingenious solutions, from which we can learn. They also give relevant feedback and advice to the services and other carers. They can also offer advocacy when needed. Carer groups are common, carer courses increasingly so. This should be encouraged. A typical course is 8 weeks and covers diagnosis, treatment, legal issues, financial issues, carers' respite and care options, how the local service works, managing expectations and free question sessions.

The carer's assessment is a right, and should be done routinely (DoH 1995). It can promote more active engagement with the service, and hopefully help retain carers after their relative has died. This is a crucial period as the carer suffers a 'second' loss, and then complex services disappear. The best practice may be to run bereavement groups to part with the service, or, better still, move on into active engagement with other carers. This will not suit all, but great experience is often lost when it could enhance a lot of what we provide.

Morbidity is high in carers (O'Connor et al. 1990; Coope et al. 1995) with high rates of depression and physical illness. This needs to be watched for in all interactions, with constant prompts to allow expression of feelings or need during every interview. For many years, these have been known to be early predictors of institutionalisation (Colerick and George 1986).

Svanberg and Stirling (1997) studied and assessed carer needs and highlighted five areas where it was felt services should improve:

- increased flexibility of day care;
- increase in community respite facilities;
- increased independent living or housing with care options;
- increased flexibility of home support services;
- more live-in companions and befriending schemes.

These need configuring in to service planning.

Summary

The changes to modernise assessment are thus:

- single referral and allocation process across all statutory agencies (integrated, care trust or otherwise);
- well developed, truly multidisciplinary CMHTs that share patient-centred aims (FMN recommendation 4; Audit Commission 2000);
- memory clinics for mild-to-moderate dementia – with standardised assessment and data collection;
- increased use of investigations, particularly imaging;
- standardised CMHT assessments for moderate-to-severe dementia;
- establishment of clear processes in the memory clinic to ensure seamless transition in to the CMHT care-managed system;
- collecting relevant health economic data as a routine;
- carers' assessments are necessary and valuable.

5 WHAT CAN THE DIFFERENT DISCIPLINES OFFER A DEMENTIA SERVICE?

The broadening out of the disciplines available in a department brings with it a wide range of approaches to any scenario and a much fuller assessment of need in any given case. It also encourages further multi-disciplinary understanding in the team, with tasks being performed by more appropriate professionals, improved recognition of relevant skills and cross-fertilisation of some of these attributes. The following sections are written by members of the Swindon service, and illustrate the added value that the therapies bring.

Speech and language therapy (SALT)

Lucy Spurway and Oonagh Wigley

Speech and language therapists (SLTs) have specialist skills and knowledge for the evaluation and treatment of communication and swallowing disorders. People with dementia are likely to have difficulties in these areas and this subsequently often leads to deterioration in quality of life for them and their carers. This section will demonstrate how SLTs therefore have an 'undeniably vital role to play in the care of the elderly with mental health problems' and are an important constituent in health-care provision for this group of clients.

The Royal College of Speech and Language Therapists (RCSLT) outlines aims and principles of service delivery in dementia in *Communicating Quality 2* – professional standards for SLTs. These are:

- to provide assessment and intervention of communication and swallowing function in clients presenting with dementia;
- to deliver services with and through carers within the client's environment as well as to the client;
- to offer advice and support to the carers in the client's environment;

- to work within a multidisciplinary framework – sharing goals of intervention and where appropriate preparing joint goals with other professionals/carers;
- to enable carers and other professionals to have a clear understanding of the communication strengths and needs of each client and provide the opportunity for the carer and other professionals to develop the appropriate skills in facilitating the client's communication.

The tremendous variation in the service provision for people with dementia in the UK is very evident in speech and language therapy, with provision varying from specialized dementia services within a community elderly mental health team (CEMHT) providing a full range of assessment and intervention to no service at all.

A report from the RCSLT working party on dementia states that elderly mentally ill (EMI) services are not seen as a priority by most districts, yet where specialist provision is available, the service is well utilized and the therapists are highly motivated, professionally satisfied and well respected.

Our experience in Swindon bears this out. Prior to 1997, there was no specialist SLT provision for clients with dementia and no links with the CEMHT. People with a diagnosis of dementia were seen within our service to adults, usually only when there was a concurrent diagnosis, e.g. cardiovascular accident (CVA), Parkinson's disease, or if there were feeding and swallowing difficulties identified whilst an in-patient on an acute hospital ward.

In 1997, resource reallocation allowed for a specialist SLT to work within the CEMHT. This role has developed over a 3.5-year period and sessions available have doubled in this time. A team of three therapists now cover 1.1 whole time equivalent (wte) sessions working within the department of old age psychiatry (DOAP).

Role of speech and language therapy

The principal role of the speech and language therapist has already been described as to provide assessment and intervention of communication and swallowing function.

Communication

Assessment

Language impairment is listed in 7.32 of the National Service Framework (NSF) for older people 2001 (Department of Health 2001a) as a feature of dementia and communication changes can often be the first sign that all is not well. Supporting differential diagnosis is therefore a key role as clients with language impairment are referred to SLT following initial assessment in the memory clinic.

Specialist SLTs have a range of formal assessments, clinical resources and knowledge relating to communication to be able to play a meaningful role in this early part of the diagnostic process. The information then provided to the Consultant Psychiatrist supplements the memory clinic assessments and supports diagnosis.

For clients with an existing diagnosis of dementia, the primary purposes of assessment have been summarized as a description of a person's communication needs, strengths and weaknesses and that person's ability to repair language and use alternative strategies when communication via spoken language fails.

Information to address the above is gathered through a variety of methods and 'communicating quality' offers advice on procedures. The battery of possible assessment types includes observation, discussion with significant others, screening, informal assessment and formal assessment.

Intervention
Once assessment is complete, the most appropriate form of intervention is planned and agreed with client and carer. These may include:

- enabling individuals to achieve maximum functional communication;
- prevention of communication breakdown between client and carer;
- education of other professionals on the nature of the communication impairments to support them in their work with the client and carer;
- monitor only;
- discharge.

Swallowing
SLTs have a significant role to play in the assessment and management of feeding and swallowing problems in clients with dementia. Specialist knowledge in the field of dysphagia can contribute to the assessment process. Alongside other relevant members of the multidisciplinary team

(MDT), SLTs can help identify whether eating and drinking difficulties result from dysphagia or are due to wider issues around dementia.

Initial assessment may lead to:

- further investigations, e.g. videofluoroscopy, ENT;
- involvement of other multidisciplinary team (MDT) members, e.g. OT, physiotherapist, dietitian, psychology, medical;
- direct SLT intervention to manage dysphagia;
- advice and support to carers on managing mealtimes;
- monitoring;
- discharge.

Conclusion

A recent report by Ponte in the RCSLT Bulletin (April 2001) compares results of a 10-year old survey of SLT services to the elderly with dementia with a repeat survey in 1999. He reports that the unmet need of 10 years ago is still present with no increase in the amount of SLT service provided to elderly mental health services in 10 years even though the elderly population has increased significantly in this time. Of 45 trusts in which no SLT services existed, 37 had no plans to develop one, even though 80% of responses indicated a need in their area.

It seems that despite SLT being identified in government reports such as the Forget Me Not report (Audit Commission 2000) and the NSF for older people with dementia (Department of Health 2001a), this client group and CEMHTs are not fully accessing specialist SLT services and subsequently not benefiting from this unique and valuable role.

Occupational therapy

Alison Warren

Theory of profession

Occupational therapy originated in North America in approximately 1917 (Creek 1997). It evolved out of theories from biological, behavioural and clinical sciences leaning towards the humanistic frame of reference (Mocellin, 1988).

The College of Occupational Therapists (1994) outline the unique core skills of an occupational therapist (OT) as:

- use of purposeful activity and meaningful occupation as therapeutic tools in the promotion of health and well-being;
- ability to enable people to explore, achieve and maintain balance in their daily living tasks and roles of personal and domestic care, leisure and productivity;
- ability to assess the effect of, and then to manipulate, physical and psychosocial environments to maximise function and social integration;
- ability to analyse, select and apply occupations to specific therapeutic media, to treat people who are experiencing dysfunction in daily living tasks, interactions and occupational roles.

Models of practice

Hagedorn (1997) clearly identified the benefit of OTs using a model of practice as it provides a map to guide the treatment process. The occupational therapy team within the Department of Old Age Psychiatry, Swindon completed an evidence-based review of models and implemented the Canadian Model of Occupational Performance (Canadian Association of Occupational Therapists 1997). This model is client-centred and uses engagement in occupation in order to promote well-being. It also has a standardised outcome measure.

To summarise, the Canadian Model of Occupational Performance states that:

- occupational performance consists of self-care, productivity and leisure;
- spirituality is the core of an individual;
- occupational performance depends on capabilities of the individual in the physical, affective, and cognitive components;
- occupational performance is influenced by factors beyond the individual, e.g. the environment or the roles one occupies;
- OTs follow a client-centred approach to practice;
- OTs attempt to promote occupational balance in order to promote health and well-being.

Development in dementia services

Historically, OTs have struggled to practise effectively in dementia care (Perrin and May 2000). OTs attempting to use rehabilitation models with this client group have often proved unsuccessful due to the deteriorating nature of dementia.

The Department of Old Age Psychiatry has benefited from a specialised and dedicated occupational therapy service since its formation in 1993. The occupational therapy team has been supported in continuous professional development and this has proven to be extremely valuable in both providing a forward-thinking service and in retaining staff. Staff of all grades also rotate between service areas, to develop skills.

Occupational therapy staff are valued members of the multidisciplinary team with clearly defined core skills and roles. Occupational therapy intervention is provided in the community, day hospital/services and in-patient settings. The development of posts working across service areas (split posts) has enabled the follow-up of clients in the community, i.e. occupational therapy intervention is initiated on the ward and continued when the client returns home and vice versa.

Changes in dementia care provision have led OTs in dementia care to develop skills in functional assessment, risk assessment (Warchol 2000) and working with carers in the home environment. The main aim of occupational therapy is not only promoting independence but also promoting well-being through the use of occupation and activity.

Occupational therapy process

The occupational therapy process outlined for the Department of Old Age Psychiatry is in line with the College of Occupational Therapists Code of Professional Conduct (British Association of Occupational Therapists 1991).

Referrals

Referrals for occupational therapy intervention are made using the department's internal referral form. There has been a steady increase in referrals, which has led to a corresponding increase in the number of OTs aligned to the Community Team within the Department of Old Age Psychiatry (Occupational Therapy Business Plan 1999/2000).

Assessment

OTs are encouraged to use both standardised and non-standardised tools during assessment, in order to both objectively and subjectively assess a client (Tullis and Nicol 1999).

Occupational therapy assessment form
The occupational therapy assessment is based on the Canadian Model of Occupational Performance (Warren 1999) and identifies client's problems/needs with activities of daily living. The occupational therapy assessment will also evaluate any changes in occupational performance.

The OT completes assessment and intervention in the three areas of occupational performance:

- self-care: personal care, functional mobility and community management;
- productivity: paid/unpaid work and household management;
- leisure: quiet recreation, active recreation and socialisation.

OTs also assess in the areas of performance components and environment as they have an impact on how an individual performs occupations.

Occupational therapy assessment tools
Allen's Cognitive Disabilities Model
The large Allen's Cognitive Level Screen (Allen *et al.* 1992) is completed by the OT to indicate an individual's cognitive abilities with activities. It enables OTs to make recommendations regarding individual needs and care planning.

Pool Activity Level (PAL) instrument
The PAL (Pool 1999) is used as an assessment tool to identify an individual's ability when completing activities. It also provides a Care Plan, which can be used by the multidisciplinary team.

Intervention
This will be on an individual or group basis, focusing on the occupational performance need.

Examples of intervention are:

- self-care: to provide equipment and advice to assist with bathing; to advise on the positioning of feeding equipment and provide adaptive cutlery;
- productivity: to provide visual cues in order to maintain skills and safety in the kitchen; to encourage and enable a client to pursue a voluntary work role;

- leisure: to introduce a client to a hobby that they value, e.g. could be a previous or new hobby; to engage a client in a sensory activity in order to promote well-being, e.g. food tasting, hand massage.

Evaluation

The final stage of the occupational therapy process involves evaluation and reflection. OTs within the Department of Old Age Psychiatry evaluate the intervention with individual clients by either using the Canadian Occupational Performance Measure (COPM) (Law *et al.* 1998) or a goal attainment framework (Occupational Therapy Audit 2001). Group work is also evaluated.

The occupational therapy process is a cycle that can be repeated if occupational needs continue to be identified for an individual that can be met by the skills of an OT.

Future developments

There are many new and exciting areas of dementia care where OTs can play a valuable role. These include:

- memory and prescribing clinic: using client- and carer-centred goals;
- introducing occupational therapy into social services/voluntary sector dementia day care;
- working in nursing homes to promote client engagement in activities;
- developing intervention shaped around the productivity and leisure needs of individuals rather than focusing primarily on self-care (Occupational Therapy Audit 2001);
- advising and supporting carers (Ching-Ching Chung 1997);
- The occupational therapy team has been instrumental in the evolution of the services for younger people with dementia in the Swindon area and will continue to be involved in its development.

The list above is not exhaustive but outlines key areas for development of occupational therapy in dementia care. All OTs working in this field have a responsibility to share ideas, innovative practice and research in order to facilitate the continued development of quality service for clients and carers.

Art therapy

Siobhan Jackson

> Art therapy provides containment during confusion, acknowledges the value of each individual ... art therapy groups can be empowering and containing at a time when body and mind are disintegrating. (Byers 1988)

This section describes what exactly art therapy is, a model that is used in the Psychiatry Of Old Age Department in Swindon with young and older people with dementia and how it can benefit this client group specifically. Few art therapists are employed in dementia services so it is a new and exciting area to be involved in. Art therapists work in different ways and this is an outline of one particular method. It is hoped that this section will raise questions for future developments and ways of working.

The development of the profession

Art therapy is a form of treatment that uses a creative process in healing (Daly 1990). Since the beginning of man, art has been used as a means of self-expression, e.g. cave paintings, Navaho Indian sand paintings, etc. As a profession, art therapy is a much more recent development, growing out of artists working in hospitals during the second world war together with psychotherapists and analysts. Today an art therapist has a first degree, usually in an art-related subject, and a postgraduate diploma in Art Therapy/Psychotherapy. It is a requirement to practice that art therapists are registered with the Council of Professions Supplementary to Medicine (CPSM).

So what is art therapy?

> The use of different art media through which a patient/client can express and work through the issues that have brought them to therapy. For many clients it is easier to relate to the therapist through the art object, which acts as a personal statement, provides a focus for discussion, analysis and self-evaluation. As it is concrete it acts as a record of the therapeutic process and cannot be denied, erased or forgotten and offers possibilities for reflection in the future. (Waller and Dally 1992)

Art therapy also allows for non-verbal communication, whereby thoughts, feelings and ideas, which cannot be expressed verbally, can be explored and contained within the image (Cox 1992). An individual can gain direct therapeutic benefit while working directly with the art media. An art therapist can provide an environment in which a patient can feel safe enough to express strong emotions, which do not have to be verbal. Therefore art therapy has a great potential to help people at every stage of their dementia.

A way of working

In the Psychiatry Of Old Age Department in Swindon, art therapy groups have been running for the last 6 months on the long stay/dementia wards and in a centre for younger people with dementia (those under the age of 65). Therefore, the treatment model used in this area is still very much under ongoing review and change.

The art therapy approach that has been found to be the most appropriate for this client group is to introduce the client or group to the art materials and gently encourage them to explore them. The patients are not formally assessed for the group as they are assessed whilst engaged in image making. The groups are 'open' patients who can come and go as they please. A non-directive approach is used, therefore, allowing the patients to make choices and decisions for themselves.

A directive approach might foster dependency, which was undesirable with patients who had already lost much independence. (Byers 1995)

Whilst engaging in image making, clients will often talk about their image, their past, or their present worries and, if the client is unable to use language, the art work can act as a form of communication. The art work is kept as a concrete reminder of the session, which can often prompt the memory of someone with dementia. Engaging a patient in the first place can be a challenge due to a lack of motivation, level of dependency and often physical needs. This difficulty can often be overcome by introducing the art materials to the client; also, the therapist's flexible approach can often capture the imagination of the client, thus enabling them to engage in image making. It has been found that drawing or painting with the client can sometimes have a positive effect. Sheppard (1998) outlines the importance of a positive relationship being built up between the art therapist and patient which is paramount when working in this area:

The relationship between the client and therapist may provide an opportunity for the person with dementia to maintain a sense of identity by counteracting social isolation or by facilitating the expression of emotion.

Art therapists can also play an important role in assessing the patient cognitive and physical levels due to observing the client interactions with the art materials (Wald 1983, 1984, 1986). The art therapist watches the client; carefully looking for the way in which images are put on the paper, it has been noticed that many clients in later stages of dementia often make disconnected images using the art materials to make rhythms on the paper, often displaying frantic mark making. Perhaps these could be linked to child developmental stages, the first stage being the scribble. Figure 5.1 shows the image of a patient in later stages of dementia who seemed to gain enjoyment from using a felt tip pen to make whirls, loops and circles.

Some benefits of art therapy

Art therapy can benefit a patient with dementia by:

- enabling the release of pent-up emotions;
- preserving the sense of pride and achievement;
- helping a patient recall past accomplishments;
- providing a non-verbal form of communication;
- recording and holding the fleeting thoughts of clients;
- enriching the experience of living long term in a hospital by providing a cultural outlet;
- maintaining a patient's identity;
- aiding the optimum functioning of remaining cognitive skills;
- fostering an environment where autonomy and choice may still be implemented.

Case study
When thinking about a case study, I thought it important to ask my clients if they would like to show their images or write a comment about their experience of art therapy. One client said he would like to show his 'tractor' images (Figure 5.2). This is what he said about his work and his experiences.

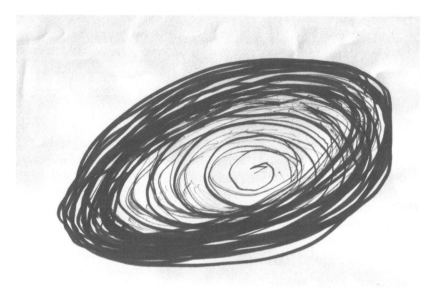

Figure 5.1   Swirls

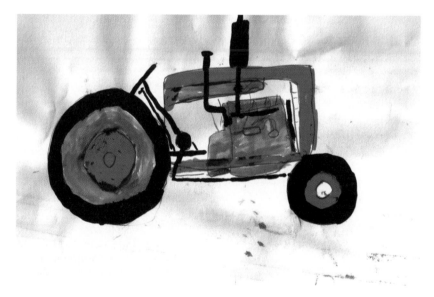

Figure 5.2   Tractor

55

I owned my own tractors in the past; I have a great love of them and used to drive and restore tractors. I enjoy coming to art therapy. I find it hard to do anything; my mind goes but when I start concentrating it's okay. A lot of the time I can't be bothered to do anything. If I don't want to do anything I won't. If there is something to do I will do it. I would describe myself as carefree, hardworking and I have a love of art. I used to be able to draw but can't now.

This client is a younger person diagnosed with 'dementia in Huntingdon disease'. He presents as a quiet person who finds it difficult to talk in groups; he also has problems with his speech due to dysarthria. At the Centre he avoids detailed creative tasks due to the frustrations they bring him. By attending art therapy this patient has had a safe space to reminisce about his past interests, which represents a time when he was stronger and more able. He talks of the present, his worries about his health and his future aims. His images are a record of this.

Recommendations for the future

It can be seen that art therapy can play an important role at both early and later stages of a person's dementia, especially as it does not necessitate the use of verbal communication. Art therapy could also play an important role in helping a younger person come to terms with their diagnosis.

Another area for development would be to use art therapy with carers' groups to help them communicate and gain support.

At the present time there is little documentation regarding art therapy practice in dementia care. More art therapists are being employed in this field, so development of treatment models, research and academic papers will be an important part of the profession's development.

Physiotherapy

Claire Leonard

Physiotherapy is a healthcare profession, which emphasises the use of physical approaches in the promotion, maintenance and restoration of an individual's physical, psychological and social wellbeing.

The profession has evolved since the Chartered society was formed in 1942. Our core skills of massage, movement and electrotherapy have been reinforced by new methods and the introduction of evidence-based practice, research and audit (Oddy 1998). The profession has seen the growth of specialist interests, with the physiotherapists acting as consultants to their peers.

Historically, in Swindon physiotherapists worked in teams providing a service to other teams, meaning they sat outside the team and had little involvement in the strategic planning or the day-to-day running. Since physiotherapists have sat directly as part of the old age psychiatry team, they are included in strategic planning and are able to educate other team members in their role. Our role in the team is to assess, advise and treat those patients with a mental health problem that prohibits rehabilitation by the acute therapists. This includes mobility problems, especially clients who are 'fallers', musculoskeletal damage, manual handling advice to carers, and education of team members to ensure clear, relevant referrals. Part of the physiotherapist's education role is to support and advise other physiotherapists in the acute hospital setting who often struggle to achieve expected goals with dementia patients.

In the early stages of the CMHT development, therapists began to care manage. This was taking up much of the therapist's workload so it is now recommended that therapy staff do not care manage as this allows them time for therapeutic interventions.

As patients are presenting with multiple pathology, in addition to their mental health problems, physiotherapists need to look at outcome measures to reflect the many differing presentations. Outcome measures are 'a test or scale administered and interpreted by physical therapists to accurately measure a particular attribute of interest to patients and therapists. It is expected to be influenced by intervention' (Mayo 1994).

Some outcome measures commonly used are:

- Tinetti Balance and Gait (Tinetti *et al.* 1986);
- Berg Balance (Berg 1989);
- Elderly Mobility Scale (Smith 1994);
- Timed Unsupported Sit/Stand;
- Functional Reach (Duncan *et al.* 1990);
- Goal Attainment scores (Kiresuk and Sherman 1968).

Outcome measures are similar to those used in elderly care and close links to the domiciliary physiotherapy service in the locality is beneficial with a clear criterion for referral to each team available. The Clinical Interest Group of Physiotherapists in Elderly Care, and the Chartered Physiotherapists in Mental Healthcare (CPMH) are both good sources of information and support in a small group of professionals. CPMH are currently looking to provide a national source book of outcome measures for physiotherapists in mental health.

Patients referred to a physiotherapist are assessed and an individualised therapeutic programme is devised by a qualified staff member. Many patients have poor balance and have fallen at least once. Following the national falls audit, therapists have improved education and assessment of 'fallers' and highlighted the need for regular assessment by physiotherapists and occupational therapists.

Technical instructors can then carry out exercise programmes on a regular basis, reviewed by qualified staff. It is often not appropriate for carers to carry out exercise programmes as this is an added stress because often patients will carry out exercises for therapists but not for carers. Alternatively, carers can become agitated and frustrated when the patient refuses to do exercises. We try and fit exercises into the normal daily activity to reduce stress and encourage near normality. Also, with a deteriorating disease, the exercises may need to be continued to prolong mobility levels.

Four good exercises to encourage all patients to do are:

- sitting unsupported for 15 minutes;
- lying as flat as possible for some time each day;
- standing supported;
- moving along the side of the bed.

Exercise groups to maintain maximum function levels and promote the importance of physical activity levels can be run in a ward setting or out in the community.

Jabadao has been shown to be of great benefit to those patients with poor cognitive function, low sensory function and high levels of personal need. This exercise is patient led, using colourful props (including beanbags, elastic rope wands and a parachute). The therapist facilitating the group will choose the music and move the group as the patients wish. Jabadao has been shown to benefit patients who do not communicate in a conventional manner. Patients who may normally sit for long periods in their own world, can for a short period be found to interact with fellow residents. Staff on the wards should be encouraged to join in these groups; carers and relatives can also join in as they can also find it beneficial.

As physiotherapists in mental health, we are concerned with improving quality of life as well as treatment and recovery (Everett *et al.* 1995). We try and establish good communication with patients, who may be unable to verbalise their feelings in a normal fashion. It is important to be able to have the skills necessary to enable a patient to feel valued. Physiotherapists are generally good at touch and can use voice intonation, facial expression, gesture and an open approach to patients. We allow them time to respond verbal or non-verbally. These approaches can, together with warm caring and reassuring handling, make a great difference to how a confused person feels.

Physiotherapists have conventional skills, but now also utilise the growing area of complementary medicine, most commonly aromatherapy and reflexology. The combination expands a lot of the non-pharmacological treatments available to patients and carers alike.

Psychology

Psychology is clearly a discipline that must contribute to the service, both in terms of assessment and intervention. It must always be remembered that older people benefit from psychological therapies as well (Wilkinson 1997). It is a hugely valuable resource, ranging from trained clinical psychologists to psychology assistants setting out towards further training – and as such, needs to be factored in to service planning (British Psychological Society 1995). Much has been written about the role of psychology in other texts, so for brevity the common services that psychology can offer are:

- assessment of neuropsychological state. This is possible using routine batteries in many dementia clinics, where other staff (e.g. nurses) often do the testing. For better interpretation of results, advice on further testing and work in multi-diagnostic memory clinics, then the presence of, or at least access to, a neuropsychologist is essential;
- work around the breaking of bad news and acceptance of the condition;

- work on memory retraining;
- combined work with the patient and carer;
- training courses for newly diagnosed patients, carers and care staff;
- psychological therapies;
- behavioural treatments;
- research.

Dietitians

The addition of a dietitian to the Swindon service showed what an important contribution dietitians can make. Audits on the wards improved staff awareness about the types and textures of food needed, and highlighted the reduced calorie intake of pureed food if given in quantities that just cover the plate. Now community assessments are leading the way towards interventions to improve diets in patients with dementia, and research into weight loss factors is starting. The relationship between diet and dementia is poorly understood, but we often see that the introduction of regular meals to our patients improves their mental state. More work needs to be done at a practical and research level, and the increased use of dietitians as part of our services can only be encouraged.

Summary points

Table 5.1 shows the contribution of the various disciplines to patients with dementia. Having other disciplines working in the dementia service brings crucial enhancement. It is important to make a commitment to developing this therapy support, as, to make it work, sensible time allocation needs to be made (not the 0.1 OT you often see allocated to a team). The workers need to feel part of the departmental team, not just a remote separate service that gets the odd referral. If integration happens, then the results are:

1) *Broader assessment* and comprehensive understanding of the patients needs. Any evaluation of a patient should take in to account six elements:
   - *contextual*: how the patient fits in what is going on around them. This needs several views and interpretations, as the context can look different depending on the observer.

Table 5.1 Contribution of various disciplines to the care of patients with dementia

Physical therapy	Occupational therapy	Speech and language therapy	Art therapy
Physical assessment	Functional assessment	Communication assessment and training	Communication with all patients with dementia
Improved mobility	Behavioural work	Swallowing assessment	Psychological interpretation
Communication via touch and movement	Relaxation	Carer strategies	Non-verbal assessments
Behavioural work	Leisure skill retraining	Managing meal times	Capturing of patient's identity
Supplying aids	Psychosocial work	Maintaining nutrition	Allowing carer expression
Relaxation and improved mood	Supplying aids	Research	Applicable in younger patients
Improved quality of life	Improved quality of life	Improved quality of life	Improved quality of life

- *difficulties*: as measured by tests. Diagnosis arises from here, but all difficulties need to be understood along with how they interact, and other disciplines collect alternative information.
- *intrapsyche*: the reaction of the individual to what is going on around them. Again, multiple perspectives are better than one.
- *effects of the past*: the more that can be gathered, from as many informants as possible, the more it helps us formulate what the person may need.
- *interpersonal skills*: are often different with different people, and the doctor especially, often gets a distorted response.
- *societal*: what the wider and immediate public make of the situation. Multiple assessments and consensus agreements minimise confusion and make the care plans more robust in the face of criticism.

2) Exposure of the patients to a wider range of specialist skills and further necessary specialist assessments. Many Alzheimer's disease patients present with communication difficulties, and aphasia needs proper assessment, as it is not always associated with dementia.
3) There is development of a *more comprehensive care plan* ...
4) ... and the team skills to deliver it.
5) *True multidisciplinary team working*: doctors and nurses with aligned social workers are not enough.
6) Reduction in the dependency on the medical model.
7) Holistic care.
8) Improved quality of life.

6 TREATMENT

The principal aim of intervening in dementia, even in the first institution-based services, has always been to maximise the independence of the individual, and help them achieve the best possible quality of life. The whole concept of quality of life and dementia is a difficult one to define, quantify, or measure, but the notion that any intervention should be aimed at producing an observable benefit is easier to work with. This benefit should primarily be for the patient, but clearly with such conditions the carer also needs to benefit, as maintaining their well-being has important consequences. The aims of all interventions should therefore be summarised as *maximising the independence of the individual, but not at someone else's expense.* If these are adhered to as basic principles, therapeutic alliances will work more productively.

The introduction of cholinesterase inhibitors in 1997 has focused the issues of treatability of Alzheimer's disease (AD) very sharply, and now NICE has endorsed their use in the NHS. Their presence is a major step forward as they have produced four effects:

- shown that a treatment does work in AD (e.g. Tariot *et al.* 2000);
- brought AD into mainstream discussion;
- encouraged people to seek help;
- shown GPs that something can be done.

But other treatment options do exist and have been used, as well as drugs. Specialist services have for some time been trying to create the opportunity to introduce them in a more proactive manner. It should also be noticed that dementia services have become very heavily biased towards AD, especially those run by psychiatrists. The 'Alzheimerisation' of dementia may have confused the issue a little, and biased our services towards preserving and substituting memory. What is becoming clearer is that core dementia symptoms relate more to loss of executive functioning, which correlates with decreasing functional abilities, which in turn predicts levels of care. A cognitive disability model is probably a more effective way of assessing all patients with dementia. This would predict levels of care, and may show up better treatment strategies than we already apply and also show us when any effort will not produce a benefit – especially in the latter stages of the disease. Cholinesterase inhibitors on the whole improve memory, behaviour and function (in clinical trials), but their effect on executive function is less clear. The nicotinic modulating effects of galantamine enhance cholinergic function and may have extra advantages (Maelicke and Alberquerque 1996).

Management guidelines have already been published (e.g. Doody *et al.* 2001). In the broader scenario of promoting independence, we can look at dementia in its stages of mild, moderate and severe and attempt to define our aims. This may also help apply resources, as although in an ideal world everybody with AD would have all possible interventions, this will be difficult to manage and sometimes completely inappropriate.

In the early stages of dementia, the aim should be to delay progression if at all possible. Such attempts may benefit the patient in gaining insight into what is happening and being able to talk about it. It would also mean that the level of disability could be stabilised for some time at an acceptable level, with the illness itself making less impact on day-to-day life. Thus, treatment here is about quality of life.

There is no clear-cut way of achieving this, but measures include:

- lifestyle changes, e.g. stopping smoking, losing weight;
- getting cardiovascular check-up, especially blood pressure;
- taking antioxidants, gingko, etc. (Sano *et al.* 1997);
- memory exercises and training;
- education about the illness for patient and carer – medical, legal, financial and issues such as driving (Lundberg *et al.* 1997);
- carers' courses (Teri 1999);
- treatment with cholinesterase inhibitors – plus any other new drugs that come into the arena.

In the middle stages of the illness, other factors come into play. Cognitive and functional disabilities need to be minimised, and emergent behavioural difficulties need treating and managing. The symptoms here are often more distressing to the carer than the patient, so the aims of intervention are different, with containing the situation a prime factor.

Measures to take here include:

- all of the above;
- symptomatic treatment with targeted interventions appropriate to the symptom and the situation;
- stabilisation of the condition where appropriate;
- more input into the carer, perhaps with programmed breaks from care and more monitoring of the carer's mental state – where intervention can delay institutionalisation (Mittelman and Ferris 1996);
- balancing the emerging conflicting needs of the patient and carer (Browning and Schwirian 1994);
- appropriate psychosocial strategies, e.g. utilising the work of Kitwood (1998);
- supporting, and not compromising the carer's role;
- ensuring all benefits and financial advice are available.

It seems apparent that when patients present at a later stage, they do less well than those who have been diagnosed earlier and progressed within a service, though no published studies prove this yet. This may be because the later presenting carers have already been traumatised and cope less well. The management here involves far more people and proper care management arrangements. One key principle at this point is ensuring *continuity of care* for the patient and carer. They need a care manager who can be called for any problem. This care manager sits between the specialist services and the primary care ones, and can either resolve a situation alone, or facilitate its resolution. The important factor for the carer is having the reassurance of someone who knows the situation in the background, who is easily available at the end of one phone call. The second key principle is that the service *does not take over care* in a paternalistic way, and thus disempower the carer, but serves to support the situation and facilitate those within it to make their own decisions (Henwood 1998).

In the final stages of the illness, the behavioural symptoms peak and then wane as the patient enters a terminal phase. The behavioural symptoms are firm predictors of institutionalisation (McShane *et al.* 1997; Kaufer *et al.* 1998), so their management at this stage is crucial if reduction, or just delay, in institutionalisation is the primary service aim. High levels of carer stress, consuming a significant amount of resource, often accompany presentation at this later stage. In some cases, the routine attempts to help maintain the case at home may prove fruitless and even detrimental. In this situation, the emotional energy can suck in a large amount of the community services time, with poor outcomes and difficult situations. Having a fast-track system to resolve these situations sensitively, usually with a nursing home placement, is a key component of a service. Often other social service departments have already been involved prior to reaching this situation, and as nursing home placement is not that specialist a process, using them to help resolve such a situation, rather than simply passing the baton on, helps maintain continuity through a difficult time. It also creates additional resource to the dementia service, whose real specialist role is helping the family understand what is happening and working through issues such as loss. Locally agreed protocols help this work.

Behavioural symptoms are a main part of current services' workload. They represent a key area where modernisation and development could take place. This is discussed further in the section on modernising current provision (Chapter 9).

What is evident from the discussion above is that there is no simple solution to each situation that presents and that what works well in one situation creates problems in another. The aim of treatment at present has to be almost biphasic:

- preservation of quality of life through information and treatment in the early stages;
- symptomatic relief and resolution of difficult situations using the CMHT and appropriate drug interventions in the later stages.

Some overlap will occur between these two aims in the middle stages, where the interventions will need to be clearly defined by the service, as it is here that often 'rationing' decisions will be made.

NICE and cholinesterase inhibitors

In January 2001, the National Institute for Clinical Excellence endorsed the use of cholinesterase inhibitors in the NHS, feeling they were both efficacious and cost-effective enough to be used. This had also been the conclusion in Canada, following a comprehensive review of the outcome measures in pivotal studies (Wolfson *et al.* 2000). Table 6.1 illustrates the main points of the NICE guidance. That the drugs work

Table 6.1 NICE guidelines, 2001–2004

- AD mild/moderate only – DLB or VaD not considered
- Severe AD has no proven benefit
- Specialist initiation only
- Need to show improvement or no decline at 2–3 months after maintenance state reached (MMSE, function or behavioural scale)
- Shared protocols can be used
- Initiate down to MMSE of 12
- People below 12 would *not normally* continue on the drugs

is no longer in question (Livingston and Katona 2000), but certain difficulties arise in the document, which affect the planning of services:

- They assume that one drug will be used for 6 months, whereas failure on one drug would normally now result in trial of another (Bullock 2001).
- They do not account for mixed dementia, which may account for up to three-quarters of what we see clinically, and has been shown to respond to galantamine (Bullock and Lilienfeld 2001). As mixed dementia is classified under AD in the ICD-10 (World Health Organization 1992), the total numbers estimated by NICE for treatment will be too low.
- They do not include patients with dementia with Lewy bodies who respond well to the treatment (McKeith *et al.* 2000) and represent 6–10% of the patients seen.
- They make assumptions about detection rates that are too low if the Forget me Not report (Audit Commission 2000) and the NSF (Department of Health 2001a) recommendations are implemented.

These four points show that all current funding estimates remain conservative and services need to plan carefully how they will meet future demand. The starting position is not good. Psychiatry as a whole only spends 1.5% of its revenue on drugs, compared with 40% in cardiology. However, 13% of all drug spending in the UK is on CNS drugs, and this is increasing. We are therefore presented with a mismatch of budgets, which arises historically from a long period of no new drug development in psychiatry (apart from antidepressants between 1960 and 1993), while at the same time sacrificing drug budgets, in order to protect services, for efficiency savings in the early 1990s. This means that every new drug that is launched is faced with scepticism, starting from the affordability angle rather than scientific argument. This should not go on, and all services should be targeted to produce drug revenues in the order of at least 10% of the total service spend. This can be done through reorganisation and reinvestment as well as new money. The services we protected in the early 1990s now have to change; therefore, starting with creating drug budgets internally in partnership with the funders is a far more mature stance than doing nothing, while asking for more.

Even with adequate changes, there will never be enough. Rationing decisions will be needed about who to treat and when. While all people with AD are entitled to treatment with these drugs, there must be a clear therapeutic aim – as, in some instances, prescribing them may make a situation worse. It is better if the treatment criteria are clear to everybody, including the patients, and that room is left to treat individuals on merit. Dogma has no place in treating this patient group. Many guidelines have already been published on how to use cholinesterase inhibitors (e.g. Lovestone *et al.* 1997; Bullock 1999) – the definitive one awaits further research.

Antipsychotics

These are commonly used in dementia even though the evidence base is quite small. It is now commonly agreed that only atypicals should be used in dementia (Jeste *et al.* 2000; Department of Health 2001a) and then only when the target symptoms are likely to respond. This has been endorsed in the NSF for older people. What this does mean is more pressure on the drug budgets and in some areas new agreements with GPs who do not like using atypicals because of the expense. These agreements are usually easy to arrange as the doses are low and the expense less obvious, but in planning a service these factors are important as not resolving them early can cause disproportionate problems. The NICE review in the second half of 2002 may help resolve the situation.

GPs in the treatment process and the issue of whose budgets

This is an issue that runs the length of the country and has different solutions everywhere. On paper, the GP's role seems clear (Downs

1996), but there does not seem a unified opinion. Dementia does challenge a lot of preconceptions and to make sense of it all means stepping aside from the traditional primary/secondary split and observing some facts:

- GPs are uncomfortable diagnosing and treating dementia.
- The responsibility for the drug and its effect lies with the prescriber.
- Patients, and the law, presume those who are prescribing understand all the possible effects of that prescription.
- Using a drug has to have a measurable benefit in terms of disease or quality of life – and be cost-effective to the prescriber.
- Most doctors rely on their own observation in making clinical decisions.
- The evidence base of new medicines involved in the treatment for dementia is changing monthly, and is barely kept up with in the specialist field, let alone primary care.
- The modern dementia services are offering almost a complete specialist primary care output already, so why split off prescribing?

These observations question what is meant by shared care protocols (e.g. in NICE). Setting up comprehensive services that may involve shared care across a number of settings is necessary. Isolating it to prescribing is going to be difficult. What doctor normally prescribes and therefore takes responsibility for all adverse events, on the say so of another service? And even if they do, what is the incentive to do so when the cost benefit lies elsewhere? Notwithstanding this view, this may become a common model of practice. I worry that this will be instead of the alternative strategy of increasing the number of memory clinics.

The best way to involve GPs in a dementia service is to use the enthusiasts as 'specialists' in the memory clinic structures, paying them appropriately and incorporating them in the learning cycles. This ensures consistency across the area in terms of practice, and assists the enthusiasts to encourage their colleagues. The treatment of dementia and the evaluation of treatment remain a specialist function in the short to medium term. Until both can be reliably performed in the GP surgery, asking GPs to pick up the cost is merely cost shunting, and it is perhaps remarkable that in some areas GPs have actually just picked up the bill as normal. I suspect that when the cholinesterase inhibitors rise to the top of the surgery pharmacy bill, the position will shift and patients may be encouraged to stop drugs early, as pharmacy data from the USA suggests – and as we see with antidepressants.

The most efficient way of dealing with this position at present is to provide the drug expenditure to secondary services, who are doing everything else, and allow them to prescribe. When and if the treatment becomes predictable enough to use simply in primary care, then the protocols that work and the budgets can be passed over together.

7 BEDS, DAY CARE AND OTHER HARDWARE

The issues around beds are complex. We started from a bed-based service and gradually lost them as time went on. Beds are an expensive resource, averaging about £30 000 each. Much of the resource released from bed closures left mental health, especially old age mental health. This occurred to such an extent that some areas have no continuing care resource at all.

The Royal College of Psychiatrists tried to stem the decline by issuing standards for bed numbers, which even at the time were probably far too high, and have not since been altered (Arie and Jolley 1982, 1998). While beds are a necessity (FMN recommendation 9; Audit Commission 2000), one of the difficulties in setting standards has been the way these services get named and how people defend what they call things to the death.

The current nomenclature seems to be that we have assessment beds, rehabilitation beds, respite beds and continuing assessment or continuing care beds, and that these mean different things to different people. Let's explore.

Assessment, rehabilitation and respite beds

These are used to admit people from the community in order to make an in-patient evaluation of what is going on. This admission may be as an emergency or planned, and is in response to not being able to manage the situation at home. In the proactive service, most of the admissions will be planned and therefore part of the ongoing community service. It could therefore be argued that this planned admission has set goals and is therefore rehabilitation – the commonest example being the treatment and resolution of a difficult behaviour. Such an admission should certainly have achievable goals, and the patient should be expected to reach discharge. In some instances the admission could even be time limited.

The emergency will become much less common, so true new 'assessment' admissions are much rarer. These, too, should have achievable goals, set within the chosen ward setting. Patients should not be fitted into any bed available, or in a totally unplanned way. If this occurs, the ward will silt up and become of little use.

It is probably best, then, to describe this bed usage as *short-term rehabilitation*. Within the health-care setting this could include respite, which should only technically be offered in a hospital to those reaching NHS long-stay criteria. Respite admissions can be used for reassessments as well as relieving the carer of burden, so it is appropriate to include them in this system. Patients who do not fulfil NHS criteria should receive respite care from the local social services, and if there is no provision, its replacement should be negotiated – the local NHS should not bale it out. What is needed is a range of respite, including emergency (FMN recommendation 8; Audit Commission 2000).

Admission to these short-term rehabilitation beds should be arranged by the community team, who set the admission goals, check they are achievable within the ward setting, and can decide the priority for admissions, based on the team feedback meetings. The consultants only need get involved in more complex risk decisions when beds are in short supply. Where there is a care manager, they still retain that responsibility through admission and liaise with the allocated primary nurse on the ward about all aspects of care, and the RMO about treatment and future care planning. If there was no care manager prior to admission, then the primary nurse assumes the role until discharge.

The 'respite' service should have a defined number of beds, to meet expected demand (Mountain and Godfrey 1995) and the process could be nurse-led. There is no need to have the patient seen by on-call junior doctors every time they come in. If a doctor is needed, this will be picked up during the nursing assessment.

Using a process like this increases efficiency, but it is difficult to predict what bed numbers are needed locally. It depends mainly on the size and style of the CMHT, but an estimate of between 0.5 and 1 bed per 1000 elderly is probably realistic.

If the term short-term rehabilitation is accepted, then the other beds can be defined as *long-term rehabilitation*. No strict time definition exists, but anything over 12 weeks is probably now a long-term prospect. This term still implies that to remain in these beds, a goal-focused therapeutic intervention is occurring, and that it is not just a care process. If this is explicit, the expectancy of a bed for life is not created, as it still means discharge is the primary aim. The entry into the longer-term beds would be via a properly set up multidisciplinary meeting involving the patient and family. This would set the goals and expectations, thus enhancing the process. Continuing care is no longer the work of the NHS – though free nursing in the care sector is (Royal Commission on Long-term Care 1999). This will require new areas of cooperation (FMN recommendation 11; Audit Commission 2000). So, while continuing assessment may be a better phrase than continuing care, it just adds to the nomenclature. The long-term rehabilitation definition has several advantages:

- It shows that the work done in dementia continues to be rehabilitation, just as seen in working with the frail elderly. As such, it is just as eligible for intermediate care as anything else. Unfortunately, it seems intermediate care has been hijacked into acute services across the UK, to the detriment of improving services for those with dementia, who most need it, especially those in the acute hospital setting. The current position should be challenged by all dementia services.
- It explains to acute services why the old 'take-away' services have stopped. Our beds exist for rehabilitation. Patients in acute services who are simply waiting for nursing homes after an accurate assessment and all rehabilitation needs assessed are no more eligible for our rehabilitation beds than theirs. This often leads to conflict over bed-blockers and fuels the assumptions that our beds are less important than the acute units. The problem actually lies usually with the hospital's admission procedures and the lack of private care home facilities. Both of these need strategic help and intervention, which our services should offer, but removal is not our task.

An interesting local finding is that many of the patients entering the local hospital in Swindon are unknown to the mental health community services, and often have a carer who has soldiered on into extremis. The commonest reasons are stigma, ignorance, or a misunderstanding with the primary care services, showing how important improving detection and referral is.

These longer-term beds should probably also be provided at a similar rate to those above – 0.5 to 1 per 1000 elderly. They *should not be mixed with older functional patients* whose needs are very different. The dementia beds should as far as possible be in purpose-built accommodation. To achieve this nationally will probably require a lot of public-private partnership, but this is appropriate, as our primary long-term aim is to provide better community services and hopefully improved treatments. Sharing the risk on accommodation is far more sensible; we do not want to end up owning a lot of empty purpose-built stock, as this would greatly reduce future financial flexibility.

One factor often not addressed in dementia services is delayed discharges and waiting times for planned admissions. The data are often collected, but do not appear in national statistics. If the waiting times for memory clinics, community assessments and placement from the community were added to our bed statistics, they would add a sizeable addition to the waiting list figures, or the new time-taken-to-be-seen tables. While old age services have prided themselves on their speed of delivery, these waits are growing in the stretched services. This needs to be made explicit – acute hospitals do very well in incentives to improve their position.

Simplifying our bed types into short- and long-term rehabilitation makes their use explicit and creates the right expectations. Similar clarity needs to be made around day care.

Day care

The need for NHS day hospitals decreases as community services expand, and in Swindon we have stopped using a specific day hospital for dementia. We do offer some day spaces on the wards for patients still at home, who meet NHS continuing care criteria, but that is all. Some day hospitals perform set assessment programmes that are comprehensive and lead to a community plan – but these assessments can all be made at the person's home. Some offer rehabilitation goals, e.g. learning to use the cooker again. This should be done at the patient's home as these skills seldom generalise. Most offer day care rather than a therapeutic intervention, and the jury is still out (Ball 1993). This should be provided by social care, not the NHS and, as stated before, if it is lacking, needs renegotiation (FMN recommendation 7; Audit Commission 2000). Day care is often best provided along with respite, and services should be able to coordinate this whether integrated or not. However, some of the individual and group work can be conducted by staff (health or otherwise) in any setting. For example, groups for newly diagnosed early-stage patients may be held in the memory clinics, while the communication groups can be in day-care centres (where other paid staff may benefit as well). But the buildings do not always need to be NHS owned.

Unfortunately, many services have day hospitals historically and fit services around them. I would contend they are relatively expensive luxuries and that expanded CMHTs offer better, more varied and more local services that deliver more appropriate and individualised care. Accepting what is inherited is not the best philosophy, and can tie up innovation and creativity for some time.

Other hardware can come from a variety of sources, mainly the *voluntary sector and the private sector.* Partnerships and innovative schemes need to be encouraged and fostered. The voluntary sector can offer service provision, e.g. home care and sitting services, advocacy and feedback. It is also often able to receive *grants from charities* such as the Lottery or Comic Relief. Useful schemes can thus be launched – the NHS need not own and control everything.

The crucial area to engage with properly is the care home sector, where the purchase of beds and joint schemes are commonplace. This topic is developed later, but a registry of good practice in this setting would be useful in order to set up local ventures.

Points to consider when setting up hardware include:

- Defining and dividing all the beds into short-term and long-term rehabilitation may simplify our stock taking and planning.
- Using rehabilitation may show the true nature of our work and qualify us for intermediate care monies.
- Careful consideration needs to take place around whether or not a day hospital is the best treatment option.
- Partnerships with the voluntary sector are crucial and can lead to innovation.
- NHS ownership of everything is both retro and potentially expensive if new treatments change the service needs of dementia patients once again.

8 YOUNG PEOPLE'S SERVICES

It is surprising that in some areas younger people with dementia have no dedicated service, or are still seen by general psychiatrists rigidly clinging to a cut-off point of 65 years (Alzheimer's Disease Society 1995). The modern dementia service sees all dementias irrespective of age, and will hopefully offer a separate system to meet the needs of this younger group.

The commonest dementias seen at this age are the frontotemporal family and AD, with a fair amount of post-stroke dementia as well. Many services also routinely accept Huntingdon's disease. These all have varying requirements, but as a group they also have specific needs (Harvey 1998). These include:

- Presentation is often with affective or anxiety symptoms and the underlying diagnosis is often initially missed. Training for GPs and generalists should be repeated often in order to raise vigilance and increase detection.
- There is often a spouse who may need to take on the breadwinning role.
- There is thus a need for a flexible day-care provision, hopefully 5 days a week.
- Patients often have relatively preserved memory so need to have directed leisure skills training to create new roles as they cease to be able to work. This is best led by therapists.
- Frontotemporal signs and symptoms need to be taught to staff and carers who may be exposed to some difficult behaviours.
- Often the families of sufferers are much younger and may require family therapy work.
- Patients and carers will need education as they will see people with different illnesses and rates of progress within the care settings, and need to understand the prognosis of their individual situation, and that of other dementias to understand what is happening to those around them.
- Many will want to discuss genetics and heritability, as these dementias are more likely to have heritable aspects. Services should know

about the genetic risks in these dementias, taking accurate genetic histories, and be cogniscent of the protocols of regional genetic services. Telling people not to worry is not reassuring or always correct. Offering evidence-based advice and using regional expertise to present choice is far more therapeutic.

- Respite services should be tailored to the younger person's needs, preferably not mixed with the very aged. Nursing home provision should be judged according to need at the time of institutionalisation – specialist homes are not always the answer.

Younger people's services are on the development agenda. Planning should be occurring across the UK to provide adequately for this group, as to date they have been poorly served. Most areas are providing new funds for such specialist services. Local providers should arrange themselves into sensible size clumps and establish units for younger people with dementia in partnership from these funds.

9 MODERNISING CURRENT SERVICE PROVISION

Clinical governance has set many challenges, one of which is to provide excellent services. As excellence is defined as something that is above average, this is impossible to achieve, as, by definition, there must be some losers (unless we are all exactly average). We now have modernisation as our new aim. Many believe they are modern enough and are unsure how to get into an improvement dialogue. A technique to help achieve this is to divide a flip chart into four squares and label them: wrong things wrong; wrong things right; right things wrong; right things right.

The task then is to brainstorm, placing all aspects of the service in one of these quadrants. Brainstorming does not allow discussion, so all suggestions are valid. This then opens up great channels for debate as several factors usually become evident. The first is that anything agreed to stay in wrong things wrong can be immediately stopped, as to continue would make no sense. In a similar way, all things in right things right should be encouraged to continue, as they will hopefully remain so. Right things wrong identifies the need for education and learning strategies to ensure maximum effectiveness. It is the wrong things right that poses the biggest challenge in the NHS. Many people are doing what they do very well and are stung by criticism that suggests they are not. It is suggesting possible alternatives that make sense, and can be owned by all, that is the major challenge in producing the change needed in order to modernise. Stopping practice is almost as hard as starting new practice, but this is where much of the resource needed to modernise will come from. For too long we have lived with the belief that old age psychiatrists provide the best for older people. While this may be true, it has resulted in the stretching of our limited resources too far. Old age psychiatry has several areas where we need to consider if current ways of working are the best. This section attempts to deal with some of these.

Behavioural problems

Behavioural problems are traditionally the entry point for many people into the dementia services, but hopefully this will be less the case as services mature – except, perhaps, in patients with dementia with Lewy bodies where the presentation is often psychiatric. Psychiatric disorders pre-empt behavioural problems and correlate strongly with carer distress and institutionalisation (Figure 9.1; Chappell and Penning 1996; Kaufer *et al.* 1998) – showing that intervention here is after the event and leaves relatively few options.

Behavioural and psychiatric disorders thus need quick and appropriate treatment. Figure 9.2 shows an algorithm to assist in treating agitation, and highlights some basic principles:

- Agitation and aggression are *forms of communication* and the *reason* needs to be established.
- *Medical problems, pain* and *drug toxicity* need to be excluded.
- *Social factors* in the patient's history may be important.
- *Environmental* or *social interactions* may be inappropriate.

To ensure that these have been thought about prior to medical inter-action, it is good practice to consider these aspects first (Bird 2000), and in the case of professional care (e.g. nursing homes) get the referrer to

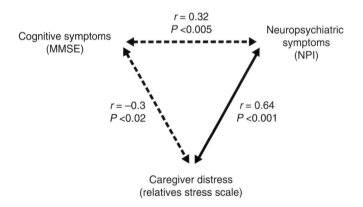

Figure 9.1   Alzheimer's disease symptoms and caregiver distress (Kaufer *et al.* 1998)

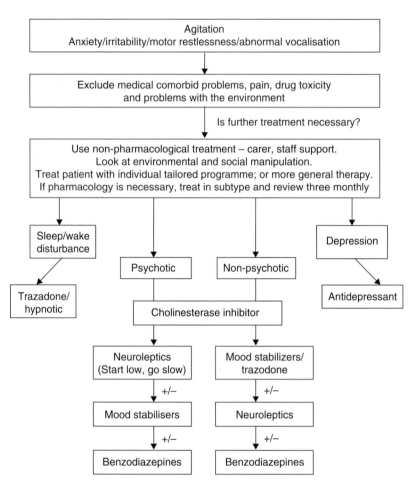

Figure 9.2   Treatment algorithm for agitation in dementia

fill in an *ABC chart*. This documents what happens leading up to the troublesome incident (Antecedent), what the problem was (Behaviour) and what happened as a result (Consequence). Using this as part of the referral process both helps the homes understand more about what their clients need (breaking the chain of dependency on local services), and reduces referral rates. This needs specialists from the community team to train the care staff, but not necessarily do all the assessments. Some

80

behaviours may then benefit from more specialised work by the team, who may have more time if the easier work is done by others. Examples of more specialised work include antecedent control, differential reinforcement or extinction.

If the behaviour requires drugs, then this is the point a doctor needs to get involved, not usually beforehand. That consultants do get involved early is often a combination of lack of available, suitable staff or protection of the DV income, both of which need addressing as part of the planning of the service. At this point the *choice of medication is really dictated by the symptoms*, applied using supporting evidence from studies on some of the drugs used in this area. What is known is that:

- Risperidone has had three positive studies in the treatment of behavioural symptoms in dementia (DeDeyn *et al.* 1999; Katz *et al.* 1999; Brodaty 2001), olanzapine has had one positive (Street *et al.* 2000) and one negative (Satterlee *et al.* 1995), so risperidone is the drug of choice in any treatment of psychotic symptoms at the current time. In this group, the antipsychotic dose is very low (0.5–1 mg risperidone), so the cost of treatment is correspondingly low.
- Cost is further reduced if patients can be reviewed at 16 weeks, as many of the behaviours are intermittent and the drugs can be stopped. This is difficult to achieve, especially if left to medical staff. Secondary care often relies on feedback from CPNs to adjust the doses; perhaps this is a sensible area to make official and use *nurse prescribing* as routine.
- Typical antipsychotics cause harm to most elderly patients, e.g. two-thirds exposed to them get tardive dyskinesia (Jeste *et al.* 1995). This suggests they should not be used unless everything else has failed.
- Consequent on the above, a *sensible addition to the drug budget* to cater for atypical use is required, and may come following the NICE decision on atypicals in 2002.
- Depression has little evidence that points to a best treatment option, though moclobemide has had a positive study (Roth *et al.* 1996) and citalopram has increasing support (Pollock *et al.* 1998). Tricyclics are very anticholinergic and should not be used, again adding pressure to the drug budget.
- Sleep disturbance responds to hypnotics and perhaps trazodone. The fear of benzodiazepines in the UK has led to some pretty toxic

Table 9.1 What behaviours respond – data extrapolated from the RCTs?

Behaviour	Risperidone	Metrifonate	Galantamine	Tacrine
Delusions	Yes	No	No	Yes?
Hallucinations	Yes	Yes	Yes	Yes
Apathy	No	Yes	Yes?	Yes
Depression	No	Yes	No	No
Agitation	Yes	Yes?	No	No
Anxiety	No	Yes	Yes	Yes
Euphoria	Yes	No	No	No
Disinhibition	Yes	No	Yes	Yes
Irritability	Yes	No	No	No
Aberrant motor activity	No	Yes	Yes	Yes

Naidoo and Bullock (2001).

choices in the past (long live the demise of thioridazine!). However, drugs like zopiclone are regularly used and provided lorazepam and temazepam are preferentially used, instead of diazepam and nitrazepam (the latter accumulate in the elderly), benzodiazepines can play a role.

- Non-psychotic behaviours have very scant evidence to support treatment choice. Many people use mood stabilisers, with valproate being popular for driven behaviours. Small studies have given some evidence, but no convincing study exists.

The best published evidence for some of these behaviours is with the cholinesterase inhibitors (Table 9.1). Galantamine reduces anxiety, wandering, apathy, and hallucinations (Tariot *et al.* 2000) in AD. Rivastigmine reduces delusions, hallucinations, apathy and depression in dementia with Lewy bodies (McKeith *et al.* 2000) and in nursing home populations has had an effect on most behaviours in two open-label studies.

So reasonable evidence supports a large area of work that occurs late in the illnesses we treat. The use of cholinesterase inhibitors remains specialist at present. But the reason I have spent so long on this section is that given this evidence, is the remaining treatment of these symptoms so complex? A large proportion of patients were treated by their GPs with thioridazine, and not referred at all – most services were only in touch with 15% of expected prevalence on average. With the evidence we have, a protocol for much of the behavioural work can be written relatively easily, and certainly with more accuracy than any shared care protocol for diagnosis and use of cholinesterase inhibitors. A protocol for treating behavioural problems would involve using the CMHT more effectively, and attempting to reduce patient exposure to drugs. We could then offer a choice between nurse prescribing (if it could be negotiated) or GP prescribing from what is clearly a limited list, starting with risperidone (ensuring somehow that cheaper, but more harmful drugs were not substituted). This would greatly reduce consultant involvement and move the chronic element of the disease towards the primary care services.

But this is a huge cultural shift. Traditionally, primary care has managed mild-to-moderate dementia, usually by attributing what is happening to normal ageing until the carers return with more explicit concerns. As a result, many referrals occur long after the shopkeeper has diagnosed the problem. Then the specialists spend 75% of their time managing moderate-to-severe dementia by propping up a failing carer – where behavioural treatments have been the mainstay of current services. Can this continue? *Maintenance of chronic illness is an area where GPs are used to working,* and protocols for this are common elsewhere in medicine, and often well accepted. As we move backwards through the illness, we must now look to hand over the more predictable parts of the illness, and stop doing what can be usefully managed elsewhere. The current vogue to cover the new workload by trying to share new services we have barely come to understand with GPs (who must understand it less) is not sensible, nor fair to the patients with dementia. The use of cholinesterase inhibitors is not in itself complex, and GPs could perform the function. But we do not fully understand how to use these compounds, and collecting systematic data now may give better protocols in the near future. I feel specialists should learn how to use these drugs properly before letting them loose in primary care. Depression is still poorly treated 20 years on, and on this occasion, perhaps patience may reap long-term dividends. When building and modernising our services, this change of who sensibly covers which part of the disease process may be a key area where we can free precious consultant time. Points to add to the service design are:

- better use of non-pharmacological techniques;
- increasing drug budgets to meet demand;

- nurse prescribing in behavioural disorders;
- changing the specialist emphasis and lessening dependence on local services;
- trying to shift the treatment of advanced chronic dementia away from specialist to primary care, with the CMHT playing a larger role between the two;
- making seeing early dementia the specialist option and using the freed up consultant time to deliver this message.

Liaison services

We know that hypertension is a major risk factor for dementia, and is often undetected or under-treated, and that altered blood rheology affects cognition. Thirty per cent of stroke patients go on to develop a dementia, and 35% of Parkinson's disease patients get depression, with similar numbers a dementia. But how many services provide formal and regular input into the acute unit provision for these problems? Most of our liaison work is advising on appropriate placements for people with moderate-to-severe dementia, advising on incapacity or protecting patients from haloperidol – and usually all fitted in on the way home. Relationships have changed with our physician colleagues, as we no longer offer the traditional take-away services we used to. This means that patients stay in acute hospitals longer than they used to; and the rate-determining step is availability of residential care options. As our services developed, geriatrics has turned to rehabilitation and stopped taking the dementia cases as well. This is a situation that needs resolving as the patients in acute hospitals suffer in clearly ageist (Lookinland and Anson 1995; Health Advisory Service 1998; Age Concern 1999) and unsympathetic (Health Advisory Service 1998; Help the Aged 2000) institutions, where discharge planning in this patient group is minimal, compared to the standards (Naylor 1994). This joint new practice could utilise intermediate care, especially where patients with resolving confusional states can gain extra time, and all services should be looking to get involved in joint schemes. If not, intermediate care will become a repository for patients awaiting care, and expectations will come on us to spend time we do not have supporting it. *Intermediate care is a new resource and should be negotiated as such.*

People with dementia have lessening verbal communication skills as the illness progresses, and so rely more on non-verbal methods.

Teaching such communication to acute hospital staff can make a big difference to how a person with dementia fares in a new setting. This facilitates a person-centred approach (Kitwood 1997), often lacking in a busy medical ward.

The assessment of capacity has been assumed to be a psychiatric role. It has also been treated as a one-off assessment. In fact, capacity is about a person's understanding at a given moment in time, and is the result of a multidisciplinary assessment convened by the RMO. In doubtful cases or those that will require the mental health act, the psychiatrist may have a role. But many cases are straightforward and can be assessed by any one who understands the criteria. A current white paper that is introducing a new *Incapacity Act* is highly bureaucratic and work intensive. It introduces the concept of the *Clinical Supervisor* who is not necessarily a doctor or the RMO. It will cover all those who lack capacity, in all health service facilities, and all residential ones. The Old Age Psychiatry services cannot take the responsibility for this within the current resourcing. We should be training all staff who deal with older people in assessing capacity now, making it clear we only need to assess the complex cases. If it is desirable for us to do more, this should be negotiated as a new service with funding to cover the time that will be needed.

Many other medical conditions have an effect on cognition, often in a subtle and less obvious way: diabetes affects executive function and slows performance. Also several commonly used medicines have a potentially harmful effect on the brain; for example, many of the commonly prescribed drugs in the elderly are anticholinergic. The benefits of setting up a *proper liaison service* instead of what seems the more *ad hoc* ones we commonly have now, may prove enormously beneficial to both patients and the acute hospitals, improving outcomes and reducing length of stay. There is currently only one full time old age psychiatry liaison post; we need to see more. Proper services need defining and resourcing, and should arguably be eligible from both intermediate care and waiting list monies.

Nursing home services

Nursing home medicine is a discipline in its own right in the USA. Here it is fitted in with the community service and run in a rudimentary fashion. Many dilemmas exist in this area:

- We know of the very high psychiatric morbidity in homes, particularly depression and cognitive impairment, but do not routinely screen or case find (Mann *et al.* 1984; Bannerjee and Macdonald 1996).
- The high exposure rates of these patients to neuroleptics, particularly antipsychotics, has been shown.
- Polypharmacy is the rule, often without reason. Structured pharmacy review may help here (Furniss 2000).
- Behavioural problems are common, but do they need consultant review? The CMHT can do a lot of this work with the GP.
- Would improved training for the nursing home staff improve the outcomes in behavioural difficulties (Moniz-Cook *et al.* 1998)?
- Have we bought in to the 'it's too late to do anything else' culture and so collude in passive neglect, aiming instead at the home dwelling?
- Would the consequences of improving quality of life at this stage make it impossible for the homes to operate on the margins they currently set?

Many more questions remain, but this is a neglected group, in spite of a college position statement 3 years ago (Jones 1998), who are currently in a private system that has all the signs of failing if radical solutions are not found. New standards are being set (Department of Health 2001b), and from October 2001 care homes and new funding streams for patients come on line. But we still compete with the private sector for qualified staff, still move the most difficult patients between various homes and the NHS. Every team still sees difficult patients turn up in their area, sometimes to homes that cannot possibly manage them, with no support.

As with other service provision, we need to negotiate a new arrangement and test new ideas (FMN recommendation 10; Audit Commission 2000). The public–private partnership scheme offers the scope to merge NHS and private cultures. We could build new facilities that were joint, abandoning traditional wards altogether, and providing care where needed. This would cut down on the movement of people as their needs change: instead more people come to them. That way all nursing would be free, and standards would rise as the nursing would be under NHS scrutiny and all therapy services would be available to all. This could get everybody out of the remains of Victorian relics into better accommodation and solve many of the dilemmas raised above.

Another theme to develop along with this would be nurse prescribing. For many behavioural symptoms protocols could be written for this to take place, especially in a setting as described. This could be a short list of allowed drugs to initiate or simple adjustment of initiated medication. Such moves would help free up consultant time for other areas, and ensure more regular reviews – and so less drug exposure for patients.

This is a difficult phase for patients and their families as it is often a terminal one, and the overall impression of going into a home is a negative one. A lot of good work and continued care management from the services helps families at this point and this needs to be more explicitly acknowledged. Work is needed to make entry into care homes a positive experience, done for good and well considered reasons – not just an end-stage phenomenon, done as there was no other choice.

In the absence of such innovative schemes, arrangements will have to be made to resource nursing home input, as local services cannot keep coping if they are net importing more difficult cases. The whole area is open for new ideas; what is clear is that this is a disadvantaged patient group that do need the NHS to take more notice.

Graduates

Old age psychiatry tends to cover all aspects of elderly mental illness, with dementia having a differing emphasis according to interest. Graduates from general psychiatry add to the workload, though should only be accepted on a case of need, not age, thus conforming with principles like choice, individualised care, care programming and professional respect. Perhaps a useful way of considering this boundary is that general psychiatry is involved with neurodevelopmental illnesses, whereas geriatric psychiatry is better equipped to deal with neuro-degenerative ones. For example, a first-time depression in a 60-year-old may be due to vascular deterioration, and would be seen as a relevant patient to the elderly service, whereas a 67-year-old with a seventh depressive illness still has their lifelong illness. Unless there is a defined reason, the latter case should remain in general services. Late-onset functional illness is an increasing speciality in its own right, with more evidence concerning the neurodegenerative aspects of its aetiology. It is impossible to work with dementia and not understand depression, psychosis and anxiety. It is possible to work on the latter and not specialise in dementia.

The boundary with adult services does need resolving in order to structure the old age psychiatry services, and their contribution to the dementia service. Younger patients with dementia need to be in the dementia services, not left where they are still commonly referred to as 'pre-seniles' because of their age. Many patients under 65 with late-onset mental illness may do better in elderly services, whereas others may not. The responsibility of the psychiatric services is to ensure that patients have an appropriate assessment, and their needs matched to the service that can meet them. The historic basis of age is clearly outdated. Protocols to agree who makes the first assessment need to be implemented, along with understanding and respect for the specialist nature of old age psychiatry. Whoever makes the first assessment identifies needs – they do not automatically 'own' the patient. The days of the RMOs arguing over who should take the patient should stop. Needs should dictate where the best care should be received, and this can be protocol led for the most part. Some informal audit work in several services has indicated that if this were to happen, the numbers of under-65s in the elderly services and the number of over-65s in the adult services would be broadly the same. If this were accepted, then any attempt to transfer all graduates to the elderly services should be seen as a new development, and properly resourced.

The common area of conflict is the elderly psychiatric rehabilitation patients. Most of these have schizophrenia, and if they develop cognitive impairment and have needs that dementia services can meet, then they should transfer. If they get frail and physical needs take over, they could go to a nursing home. What they should not do is go to a dementia ward because they are 65. This is grossly unfair to them and the patients with dementia – the groups should not be mixed. If a resource is needed for these elderly graduates it should be negotiated as a new service, and as the numbers are small, probably on a partnership basis with other trusts.

Conclusions

- These four areas (behavioural problems, liaison services, nursing home services and graduates) make up a large proportion of our work; two could be done by others, two need appropriate funding to be done properly.
- New core work needs defining and assigning properly.

- New boundaries need renegotiating.
- This would enable a redistribution of some existing resources.
- It would also clarify expectations and dispel old myths.
- Proper costing of what we are capable of offering may lead to better funded services.

10 NEED FOR DEMENTIA SERVICES – BETTER DELIVERY, BETTER GOVERNANCE, LESS VULNERABILITY

A fundamental problem in building a dementia service is that the concept as such does not actually exist. People suffering with dementia may be seen by a psychiatrist, a geriatrician or a neurologist (usually younger patients) for their initial assessment. All offer comprehensive diagnostic procedures and most offer treatment, but only the psychiatry services tend to offer access to multidisciplinary ongoing care.

Likewise, few guidelines exist on the treatment of dementia (Eccles *et al.* 1998; Naidoo and Bullock 2001) and these do not address the need to set up specialist services.

To date, the services that old age psychiatry provide have not been so clearly defined. They have become larger and incorporated more, often in the fervent belief (often true) that they offer the best service to this patient group. It is now difficult for the single old age psychiatrist to perform all the roles with which they are currently invested. The National Service Framework for Older People has helped clarify things in some ways, but not helped in others. It sends a fairly clear message that older people's services need to align more and integrate in certain ways, moving us away from the traditional resting place in mental health. It sets targets for the services (Table 10.1), with timescales that are perhaps disappointingly long. It also helpfully clarifies the importance of memory clinics and states older patients with dementia should receive newer antipsychotics – upholding the direction our practice has gone. What it has not done is offer new resources, maintaining that they may already be there. Whilst this may have an element of truth, new investment may have stimulated a better response, and not cast some doubt about intention. Two ironies present: *dementia care is provided for by the least resourced services, even though it is the most expensive disease; but also, not investing in elderly services could be construed as discriminatory, something the NSF is at pains to root out.*

Table 10.1 NSF standard seven: mental health in older people

Aim
To promote good mental health in older people and to treat and support those older people with dementia and depression

Standard
Older people who have mental health problems have access to integrated mental health services, provided by NHS and councils to ensure effective diagnosis, treatment and support, for them and their carers

Milestones – by April 2004
- HImPs and other relevant local plans developed with local authority and independent sector partners, should have included the development of an integrated mental health service for older people, including mental health promotion
- PCG/Ts will have ensured that every general practice is using a protocol agreed with local specialist services, health and social services, to diagnose, treat and care for patients with depression or dementia
- Health and social care systems should have agreed protocols in place for the care and management of older people with mental health problems

A summary of what each standard of the NSF means to old age mental health services is shown in Table 10.2.

The Forget Me Not report (Audit Commission 2000) highlighted the resource issue. Using the centres chosen, it gave a UK average spend per head of elderly population of £80. This can be used to calculate where a service may be, and what the expectations really are with current funding. For example, the Swindon old age psychiatry service (NHS part) provides for 29 000 people, meaning it should receive £2.3 million pounds to reach average; like many others, it does not.

It may therefore be necessary to more clearly delineate the dementia components in order to use them more efficiently and protect them (FMN recommendation 12; Audit Commission 2000). Old age psychiatry has been the most vulnerable part of mental health and remains so following the NSF for older people. Dementia is a lower priority in geriatrics and resources get lost in the rehabilitation agenda. Neurology will diagnose, and possibly treat in some areas, but offers no holistic continuity. GPs come into contact with dementia on a haphazard basis, except for some notable enthusiasts. Social services often do not have specialist elderly care workers. This disparate use of resource needs to

Table 10.2 How the Older Persons National Service Framework (NSF) impacts on old age psychiatry and dementia services

Standard 1, Age discrimination	Mental health services should not be age specific, so the elderly are entitled to services in this and the mental health NSF
Standard 2, Person centred care	This applies in mental health issues as well, so single assessment processes must contain the relevant information
Standard 3, Intermediate care	Applies to mental health as well. Rehabilitation should be offered for depression and cognitive disorders to reduce hospital stays and early care home placement
Standard 4, General hospital care	Specialist care should be available in hospitals where diagnosis of depression and dementia are crucial, and properly thought out ward environments may help the confused. Such increased service needs resource
Standard 5, Stroke Standard 6, Falls	Overlaps with dementia and depression – joint services to be encouraged Depression and dementia increase the risk of falls, and correct use of many drugs, especially psychotropic is important
Standard 7, Mental health	Highlights need for early diagnosis of dementia Need integrated community services, better detection of mental illness, improved communication between agencies and new measures in nursing homes States tricyclic antidepressants and atypical antipsychotics are preferential choices in older people Suggests there is a place for psychotherapy
Standard 8, Medicines	Reduce polypharmacy, increase reviews and use more antidepressants if appropriate Care homes need more training in non-pharmacological methods

be pulled together in each area, and a defined resource for treating dementia pooled and arranged to deliver services based on the content of the previous chapters.

If we do not create dementia services in geographically defined areas, gains in efficiency from economies of scale will not be made, resources will be lost, and sensible care pathways and agreed treatment centres will not be set up. It is not the 'who' that is the issue in setting up these services – so long as workers are enthusiastic, able and committed. The important thing to agree is the 'what' and the processes that will deliver it.

What organisation meets the needs?

The ideal dementia service may be best set up as a virtual entity, existing as a well-organised set of processes across several organisations. An example of this that has worked well is the drug action teams, which have identified and ring fenced resources across a range of organisations, both statutory and voluntary, and created very effective care systems. This model would allow rapid progress and minimal disruption. Unfortunately, such collaboration is rare, as different organisational pressures strain these relationships, and concentration on structure rather than function is the norm, especially in today's ever-changing world. It also seems rare that old age psychiatry services even know what their budgets are – something that needs to be rectified as a priority. However, the newly developing cancer collaboratives are gaining acceptability, so may help establish this as a more accepted model of working.

In Swindon we have formed the basis of a Dementia Action Team, building on the drug/alcohol work and the cancer collaboratives. This will be based from the primary care trust (PCT) and run as a virtual organisation, aiming to identify all resources and restructure services accordingly. This work will continue over the next 3 years, and result in dedicated dementia services within a new older peoples directorate.

Where do dementia services fit?

If the dementia service is going to be housed in a single organisation, how can we decide which is best?

- Older people's services are being united in the NSF, implying a strategic move towards *integration of old age psychiatry and geriatric medicine,* which makes a specialist mental health trust an unlikely host.

- The service has a large *community* component, which suggests that an acute trust is far from ideal.
- Integration of old age psychiatry and social services has been occurring over the last few years and *care trusts* are now emerging after the Health Act, making the PCT or mental health trusts more likely.
- The assessment process involves a lot of acute hospital facilities, e.g. imaging, though this has not been a problem to date.
- Shared services with primary care may best take place in a primary care organisation. This is especially true for shared care protocols that involve prescribing new drugs. Figure 10.1 shows some of the organisational options. The economic models predict new drugs may be cost neutral, but this assumes one system, where social care savings are released back to fund medication. The only single organisational way this can occur is in a *PCT care trust.* Without this, no GP is going to agree to fund social services savings.

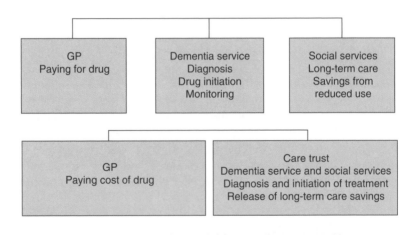

Figure 10.1 Options in providing cholinesterase inhibitors

- The dementias are not mental illnesses, they are a set of physical conditions with psychiatric features as a part of the syndrome.

Keeping with the principle it is the 'what' rather than the 'who' that is important, an effective and *well run collaborative model* should be the most exciting ideal, and would logically be hosted in the PCT. The important dimension for dementia services is to ensure that the monetary aspects flow through the system, and are kept within it. If this occurs sensible care protocols will come out of the process, with the most appropriate person doing the most appropriate task. As things currently stand, shared care often relates to shared expense and cost shifting, rather than cost-effective patient care.

Secure foundations for building a dementia service can be obtained by:

- identifying your own budget, and calculating the average spend based on the FMN report – then comparing;
- identifying all the local existing resources being used for dementia;
- arranging them systematically to see where there are gaps and if there is duplication;
- considering the prospect of setting up a formal dementia collaborative;
- deciding how this combined service will relate to existing services;
- choosing the most appropriate organisational base from which to work – which appears to be the PCTs as they become established, either as collaborative host or defined organisation.

Managing complex situations

It is clear that modernising dementia services in the current climate is a complex task. In this situation, the temptation is to try and write a huge plan and then rigidly implement it. The field of dementia is changing. Plans written 5 years ago would be obsolete, as symptomatic treatments have been introduced over the last 4 years. In 5 years' time, we may have disease modification that will render this year's plans obsolete. What we need is a sensible strategic direction with enough fluidity to develop according to changing developments and need. This will need flexible management techniques that are not so reliant on the rules of certainty – the situation we keep coming up against today as services centralise and stiffen.

Simple rules

Many feats of nature occur through inherent order that allows them to happen. For example, flocking birds do so without a squadron leader, but by following three rules: when you see a flock, fly close to another bird, match their speed, and move to the centre of the mass of birds. These rules allow a complex phenomenon to occur, one so complex that a computer cannot generate it (no 500-page plan can give the answer), unless it, too, programmes in the same rules.

Services can adopt the same principles, setting simple rules to its staff to encourage innovation and learning. This will involve trial and error, so the rules must protect patients. This can produce huge strides without the need for complex planning, and helps staff own the changes.

Bold aims

Simple rules have to have a strategic context. This will be set by national and local imperatives. The duty of the strategic management is to put forward strategic goals, in the form of bold aims (FMN recommendation 15; Audit Commission 2000). These need to be adventurous yet realistic, involving everybody in achieving them. A relevant example would be to reduce nursing home placement by 10% in 4 years. This is a bold aim with many routes to implementation. Setting simple rules will throw up many attempts at these routes, some of which will work, whilst others will fail. Failure and error are thus learning processes, which if properly managed are a necessary and integral part of development and management in a complex situation – not problems, as often it seems to be how they are viewed. Oscar Wilde correctly proclaimed, 'experience is the name we give to our mistakes'. Thus a large step can be made possible through many incremental and coordinated steps, which occur as an ongoing process (the true meaning of strategy), not through a large planning document.

Incremental steps and large contextual leaps are productive methods of change and when combined together are synergistic. Some further examples of simple rules and bold aims are in Table 10.3. As a

Table 10.3 Simple rules and bold aims

Simple rules	Bold aims
• Stop waiting to be told what to do • Identify all resource and use it • Problem solve, not generate • Look at what best practice you can build around your patients • Work with neighbouring colleagues to provide care as a group – not necessarily all yourself • If it goes well, tell us. If it goes wrong – stop, work out why and tell us • Collect simple outcome data	• All services integrated • Seamless services in/with primary care • 66% detection rate of AD in 5 years • 66% of that detection in mild (and early moderate) illness • Care home EMI placements down by 15% in 5 years • Basic pharmacology routine in OAP in 3 years • AD a primary care disease in 10 years

management philosophy, this is applying clear leadership without the need for complex structure, especially if across numerous organisations. Setting common philosophies allows development while empowering staff and maintaining the identity of members of the collaborative. This offers a simple process through the undoubted complexity.

Managing the dementia service entails:

• agreeing a common set of philosophies and standards across all those involved;
• using these to create some bold aims;
• setting simple rules for the staff, in order for them to work to bold aims;
• allowing trial and error within these rules;
• creating good information systems to follow the work – FMN recommendation 16 (Audit Commission 2000);
• keeping plans, policies and procedures to an absolute minimum;
• remembering this is an evolving field, so services need to be able to evolve with it – FMN recommendation 17 (Audit Commission 2000).

Steps on which to build services

Every system is perfectly designed to deliver the result it gets. If the service is good, then it is probably designed well. If the current service is not working well, it is the current service that needs to change – too often lack of development is openly blamed on those above or outside the organisation imposing restrictions; or those below not being ready for change. These rationalisations are barriers and implicitly protect the status quo. What is wrong needs to be identified long before more resources are demanded to fix the problem; *more money thrown at the wrong system will not help it*, just create a larger mess. Bearing this in mind, the first step is to run a needs assessment across the service to see where it is lacking or causing worry.

To do this, *national and local expectations need to be fully understood* and incorporated into planning. In addition, taking a long-term view helps to predict future priorities before they are declared. This causes less disruption to service and leaves everybody feeling they are more in control of their destiny.

Everybody must realise that they play a role in the delivery of patient care within the system in which they work. They must understand that role and stick to it, and appraisal is the tool to assist this. This includes the consultant, who should be appraised by the service as well as the medical managers.

Virtual collaborations should be built so local resources are understood. This will go some way to clarifying what the task is. This pooled resource could develop into the dementia collaborative of the future, and be a major step in modernisation.

The gaps should be established and some of the ideas in this text used to overcome them, whilst adding alternative ideas in locally sensitive plans. This should involve all who contribute to the service, including patients and carers and GPs, who, if they own the services more, will protect and support their stability and free them from any sudden changes or decisions.

11 DEVELOPMENT THEMES FOR MODERNISATION OF OLD AGE PSYCHIATRY SERVICES

A consensus statement from the World Health Organisation and the World Psychiatric association (World Health Organization 1998) set out some principles for care of older people with mental illness. With some minor changes from the original, Table 11.1 sets out these principles, so as to prove that old age psychiatrists do it with charisma.

Principles of care in modern services

The following principles are essential in the underpinning of our services as they undergo the necessary re-engineering to meet the changing demands of our profession. To lose sight of one would compromise the system that they all configure:

- paramount focus on the clinician–patient relationship;
- individualised access to care and information at all times;
- knowledge-based care is the standard;
- individuals control their own care to the extent that each individual desires;

Table 11.1 WHO/WPA consensus guidelines on the qualities that make up mental health services for older people. Or 'old age psychiatrists do it with....'

- Comprehensive
- Holistic
- Accessible
- Reliable
- Individual
- Sustainable
- Multidisciplinary
- Accountable

- minimal waiting for all involved in the processes of care;
- seamless transfer and communication of information and coordination of care;
- financial performance sufficient to ensure unhindered quality;
- patient and practice management based on real-time data, including measures of process, satisfaction, finance, outcomes and epidemiology;
- continual improvement and waste reduction in all processes and services;
- individual health linked to broader community health;
- a model work environment.

These principles will ensure patient-focused care in a newly created culture where continuing development of services based on regrowth as well as new investment becomes the norm. Our current culture can then move to one of enquiry and change, as these principles will drive that for as long as they are applied. Once the culture changes, good facilitation can bring about effective implementation of evidence and introduction of new methods.

In order to implement the principles, four themes need to be addressed as pillars on which to benchmark and plan change. These four themes are patient based, involving their journey through a contact with the care system, ensuring that development occurs at points relevant to patient care, making sure patients, not the service, are the beneficiary of any change. These themes are:

- access
- interaction
- reliability
- vitality.

Access: the help I want and need when I want and need it

- Timing of care entry needs to be made specific for dementia care pathways
- Care is not just about encounters or visits – the patients need to feel that the specialist service they receive is ongoing
- Care involves access to information, support, dialogue, reassurance and treatment

- Services need to provide 24-hour, 7 days a week, 365 days a year access
- Open access scheduling to meet varying demand and emergencies; nurse-led clinics and leaving open slots in out-patient department schedules are good practice examples
- Non-visit care models; phone response or interactive web-based problem solving
- Self-care groups, facilitated by the specialist services both for carers, and as diagnosis occurs earlier, patients as well
- Group visits/waiting room training methods, e.g. carers' courses covering topics such as medication, benefit briefs
- Prediction planning for the individual case (e.g. contingency planning for frail relatives) and disease prediction for the individual and the local population
- Huddles and patient panels to inform quality issues and provide advocacy
- Real-time on-line reallocation of resources to aid improvement in access

Outcome measures
- Time until next appointment and the time until the third next available appointment
- Future capacity – total available appointment time over next 4 weeks
- Team patient match: % patients seeing their correct care team
- DNA rates
- Volume of use of non-one-to-one visit services (e-mail, groups, web)
- Patient ratings of access to services

Interaction: the help I want and need when I want and need it
- The ideal interaction equates to idealised care
- Customisation of the style and timing of communications
- Staged delivery of information in order to break bad news effectively at the patient's pace
- Shared decision making
- Coaching and written information about visits, so that the patient knows what to expect and how to get the best out of the interaction

- Patient self-management systems
- Compliance is about communication; non-compliance is not the patient's fault
- Team training in communication skills
- Patient-owned records and patient-held notes
- Short cycle of evaluation of all reports and tests
- Transparency for all laboratory and test results
- Web-based care and information
- E-mail to patients and carers where appropriate
- Creation of disease registries, especially for at-risk groups

Outcome measures
- Clinician–patient match
- Patient report of visit benefit
- Patient satisfaction with explanations about problems treatment and general health improvement
- Number of patients and carers/month using interactive technology

Reliability: exactly the help I want and need when I want and need it

- Use of registries and proactive population management
- Master rescheduling of resources to where all agree they are now needed
- Systems incorporate new science whenever it becomes available
- Adoption of best practices: protocols and guidelines
- Graphical representation of practice measures of progress and outcomes
- Surveillance for under- and overuse of interventions
- Blame-free error surveillance (good practice is not error free)
- Adverse event recording: using better capture mechanisms than simple voluntary reporting
- Remembering that discharge is not an event: transfer to other care is part of an ongoing process
- Fail safe systems for bringing patients into care when necessary
- Coordination across boundaries
- Reducing cost by removing waste
- Safety systems and fixed responsibility for safety oversight
- Tell quickly when hypotheses fail in order to both change and learn

- Systems for coordination with outside inspection/consultancy to facilitate the visits and ensure dissemination of learning from them

Outcome measures
- Hospitalisation rates per team
- Emergency/urgent care rates per team
- Disease-specific health outcomes
- Conformance of care to agreed protocols
- Reports on safety conditions and hazards
- Percentage of patients assessing continuity of care as good or excellent

Vitality: they can give me exactly the help I want when I need it

- Sustainable redesign processes
- Continual innovation and improvement
- Innovative planning systems: most will come from understanding of need, not from the patients asking directly
- Research and development
- Staff development systems
- Processes for forming strategic alliances
- Smart business sense
- New resource through waste reduction
- Wise investment
- Innovative payment systems within the NHS constraints
- A service that surprises people and remains unpredictable

Outcome measures
- Patient number on books
- New patient visits/month
- Volume of non-one-to-one visits provided
- Margin on the yearly budget
- Staff morale

These principles apply across race and creed. I have not talked specifically of ethnic minority services, but would say that individualised services should meet individual needs. This means that cultural awareness has to be part of ongoing staff development, ensuring special situations are recognised. In areas where there are high numbers of certain ethnic groups, then a properly conducted needs assessment should indicate the requirement for any particular special service. Some prevalence studies offer clues as to the numbers of ethnic elders who are at risk (Brownlie 1991; Silveira and Ebrahim 1995; McCracken *et al.* 1997).

12 FUTURE DEVELOPMENTS

Dementia services pose challenges now. But what does the future hold?

I think we will continue to move on backwards through the illness as we learn more. Mild cognitive impairment is already being diagnosed (Peterson *et al.* 2001) and studied, and we have opened our first mild memory disorder clinic in Swindon. We will all become clearer about aetiology and differential diagnosis, and learn to look at dementia as more than just AD. This will make it possible for treatment before the worst symptoms appear, with further reduction in the severe cases and better use of the resources we have. Cure is still a wish for most medical problems, not just dementia, but disease modification and containment is common and this looks possible for AD (and perhaps some other dementias) in the not too distant future. When this occurs, the earlier the intervention the better.

We already know from positron emission tomography (PET) studies that some of the changes to nicotinic receptors are occurring 12 years before symptoms appear, that magnetic resonance imaging (MRI) scans show hypothalamic atrophy prior to significant symptoms and that long-term hypertension is a predictor of both vascular dementia and AD (Forette *et al.* 1998). Whilst PET scanners are still research tools, MRI has become less expensive and even functional imaging is available in some general hospitals. Measuring the brain volume change (Fox *et al.* 2000) may thus become a standard biomarker over the next few years, and help with earlier diagnosis.

We have seen that oestrogen (Tang *et al.* 1996), non-steroidal anti-inflammatory drugs (McGeer *et al.* 1996; Mackenzie 2000) and statins (Jick *et al.* 2000) may have a protective effect, lowering the risk of dementia after long-term use. How and why this is so is not yet fully understood, but elegant models offer some explanation and ongoing trials will yield more information.

Genetics continues to reveal more about the dementias. ApoE4 is a known risk factor in AD and several genes have been identified for early AD. Whilst our knowledge at present is rudimentary, further clarification will occur as methodology improves. Genetic screening is currently not part of our work, but knowledge of it is necessary and it may become so as more is understood (Post *et al.* 1997).

All these factors contribute to the concept that we develop 'brain failure' as we grow older, and that part of a dementia service's role will be to work more with physicians in *optimising brain protection* throughout a person's middle-to-late life. The memory clinics may expand to incorporate a 'well-brain' clinic that offers a check on risk factors, medication and blood pressure for people from 50 onwards. Such a public health function may actually have as much effect on the reduction of severe dementia as drug therapy post-symptoms.

Such clinics offer a role for specialist nurses, who will also hopefully be able to take on a limited prescribing role. This continues to have a direct effect on consultant time, in freeing it up in some areas to refocus it on newer services, a situation that will hopefully be complemented by increase in numbers.

We should perhaps become more proactive at following up our known at-risk populations:

- mild cognitive impairment
- post-stroke
- post-confusional episodes
- pseudodementia
- Parkinson's disease.

These patients should be placed on *case registers* and followed up for signs of increasing cognitive impairment, even if only with a simple test or a telephone system (Carpenter and Strauss 1995; Gatz *et al.* 1995). This could be true shared care with the primary care services. This would facilitate the early detection of cognitive decline and lead to possible early intervention, and remove some of the hurdles that delay detection.

Drug treatments will continue to develop. There is already an amyloid inoculation in development (Schenk *et al.* 2000) and now specific enzyme blockers for pathological processes in AD. As a magic bullet treatment is unlikely, *combination therapy* will undoubtedly occur – as it does in most chronic illnesses. Services need to ensure that they remain *up to date with emerging pharmacology,* and are *strategically creating budgets* to do so. This means continual reinvestment of any savings within the system, and bidding for any funding that is relevant to creating new services.

Drug development and neuroscience research is giving us exciting times, but some simple compounds such as folate or vitamin E also show some potential. What will be needed as time goes on will be *larger trials* to show true epidemiological effects, and whether these are affordable remains to be seen. They will need central funding as some questions will not be of interest to pharmaceutical companies, so hopefully the *MRC and perhaps the European Union will take more interest.* Perversely, new developments in drug technology could outstrip available resource, even in the pharmaceutical industry, if we are not careful, and all the advantages of our move forward could be compromised.

This all suggests that the future role for dementia services will be to move towards *primary prevention* as well as treatment. Much of what we do now may end up in what is now primary care, as may our services. The work specialists currently do now may well change significantly, but there are new and exciting opportunities with which to replace it. There actually is hope that over the next 20 years we will see major advances in the treatment of dementia, especially AD, and subsequent wholesale change of the services needed. *If this led to the significant reduction in the numbers of those reaching the severe dementia stage, along with a lessening of the stigma of this disease, then we would have contributed to and witnessed a major medical and social phenomenon during the course of our careers.*

Modernising and building services that are fit for purpose, and equitable across the UK is the first stage in achieving this remarkable goal. Looking at what we currently have, followed by repatterning of services is the first step to do this, and the environment is right. Creative thinkers need to be encouraged now, and the local organisations need to strive to make the dementia service a reality. Patients deserve this and it can be done.

Let's stop talking about it, let's not write long strategic plans – LET'S JUST DO IT!!

That just leaves the real challenge, which has existed for many years and continues to remain unresolved: when are we going to be able to come up with an effective name for the services we work in, which attracts people, makes it clear what is on offer and does not scare people off?

I have always liked behavioural neurology, but accept its limitations – all suggestions to:

roger.bullock@kingshill-research.org

REFERENCES

References marked with a diamond (◇) in the margin are key references.

Age Concern (1999) *Turning Your Back on Us. Older People and the NHS*. Age Concern, London.

Allen CK, Earhart CA, Blue T (1992) *Occupational Therapy Treatment Goals for the Physically and Cognitively Disabled*. The American Occupational Therapy Association, Inc., USA.

Alzheimer's Disease Society (1994) *Home Alone: Living Alone with Dementia*. ADS, London.

Alzheimer's Disease Society (1995) *Services for Younger People with Dementia*. ADS, London.

Aneshensel C, Pearlin L (1995) *Profiles in Caregiving: the Unexpected Carer*. Academic Press, London.

Arie T, Jolley D (1982) Making services work: organisation and style of psychogeriatric services. In: Levy R, Post, L (eds), *The Psychiatry of Late Life*. Blackwell, Oxford.

Arie T, Jolley D (1998) Psychogeriatric services. In: Tallis RC, Fillit HM, Bocklehurst JC (eds), *Textbook of Geriatric Medicine and Gerontology*, 5th edn, pp. 1567–73. Churchill Livingstone, Edinburgh.

Askham J (1995) Making sense of dementia: carers perceptions. *Ageing Soc* **15**, 103–114.

◇ Audit Commission (2000) *Forget Me Not – Mental Health Services for Older People*. Audit Commission, London.

Ball C (1993) The rise and fall of psychogeriatric day hospitals. *Int J Geriatr Psychiatry* **8**, 783–4.

Banerjee S, Macdonald A (1996) Mental disorder in an elderly home care population: associations with health and social service use. *Br J Psychiatry* **168**, 750–6.

Bannerjee S, Dickinson E (1997) Evidence based healthcare in old age psychiatry. *Int J Psychiatry Med* **27**, 283–92.

Berg K (1989) Measuring balance in the elderly: preliminary development of instrument. *Physiother Can* **41**(6), 304–11.

Bird M (2000) Psychosocial management of behaviour problems in dementia. In: O'Brien J, Ames D, Burns A (eds), *Dementia*, 2nd edn. Arnold, London.

Black SE, Blessed G, Edwardson JA, Kay DWK (1990) Prevalence rates of dementia in an ageing population: are low rates due to the use of insensitive instruments? *Age Ageing* **19**, 84–90.

◇ Bosanquet N, May J, Johnson N (1998) Alzheimer's disease in the UK: burden of disease and future care. *Health Policy Review Number 12*. Imperial College of Science and Technology, London.

British Association of Occupational Therapists (1991) *Code of Professional Conduct.* College of Occupational Therapists, London.

British Psychological Society (1995) Purchasing clinical psychology services, services for older people, their families and other carers. *Briefing Paper No. 5.* BPS, Leicester.

Brodaty H (2001) The results of the RIS-AUS-3 Study. Presentation at the 10th IPA Congress. Nice, France.

Brooke P, Bullock RA (1999) Validation of a six item Cognitive Impairment Test with a view to primary care usage. *Int J Geriatr Psychiatry* **14**(11), 936–40.

Brookmeyer R, Gray S (2000) Methods for projecting incidence and prevalence of chronic disease in the aging population: application for Alzheimer's disease. *Stat Med* **19**(11–12), 1481–93.

Brookmeyer R, Gray S, Kawas C (1998) Predictions of Alzheimer's disease in the United States and public health impact of delaying onset. *Am J Public Health* **88**(9), 1377–42.

Browning J, Schwirian P (1994) Spousal caregivers burden: impact of care recipient health problems and mental status. *J Gerontol Nurs* **March**, 17–22.

Brownlie J (1991) *A Hidden Problem? Dementia Amongst Minority Ethnic Groups.* Dementia Services Development Centre, University of Stirling.

Bullock R (1999) Drug treatments for early Alzheimer's disease. *Adv Psychiatr Treat* **4**, 126–34.

Bullock R (2001) Switching cholinesterase inhibitors – is it worth it? Poster at 10th IPA Congress. Nice, France.

Bullock R, Lilienfeld S (2001) Galantamine shows promising results in probable vascular dementia and Alzheimer's disease with cerebrovascular components. Poster at 17th World Congress of Neurology, London.

Byers A (1988) Candles slowly burning. In: Skaif and Huet (eds), *Art Psychotherapy Groups*, London.

Byers A (1995) Beyond marks – on working with elderly people with severe memory loss. *Inscape* **1**, 13–18.

Canadian Association of Occupational Therapists (1997) *Enabling Occupation: an Occupational Therapy Perspective.* CAOT Publications, Ottawa.

Caro JJ, Getsios D, Migliaccio-Walle K, Raggio G, Ward A for the AHEAD study group (2001) Assessment of health economics in Alzheimer's disease (AHEAD) based on need for full-time care. *Neurology* **57**, 964–71.

Carpenter B, Strauss M (1995) Telephone assessment of memory in the elderly. *J Clin Geropsychol* **1**(2), 107–17.

Chappell N, Penning M (1996) Behavioural problems and distress among care givers of people with dementia. *Ageing Soc* **16**, 57–73.

Chew CA, Wilkin D, Glendinning C (1994) Annual assessments of patients aged 75 years and over: views and experiences of elderly people. *Br J Gen Pract* **44**, 567–70.

Ching-Ching Chung J (1997) Focus on family caregivers for individuals with dementia: implications for occupational therapy practice. *Occup Ther Int* **4**(1), 66–80.

Clarfield AM (1988) The reversible dementias: do they reverse? *Ann Intern Med* **109**, 476–86.

Colerick E, George L (1986) Predictors of institutionalisation among care givers of patients with Alzheimer's Disease. *J Am Geriatr Soc* **34**, 493–8.

College of Occupational Therapists (1994) *Core Skills and a Conceptual Framework for Practice.* College of Occupational Therapists, London.

Connell C, Kole S (1994) Increasing coordination of dementia service delivery network: planning for the community outreach education programme. *Gerontologist* **34**(5), 700–6.

Coope B, Ballard C, Saad K *et al.* (1995) The prevalence of depression in the carers of dementia sufferers. *Br J Psychiatry* **10**, 237–42.

Cox M (1992) *Children's Drawings.* Penguin Books, London.

Creek J (1997) *Occupational Therapy and Mental Health.* Churchill Livingstone, London.

Daly T (ed.) (1990) *Art Therapy – an Introduction to the Use of Art as a Therapeutic Technique.* Routledge, London.

DeDeyn PP, Rabheru K, Rasmussen A *et al.* (1999) A randomised trial of risperidone, placebo and haloperidol for behavioural symptoms of dementia. *Neurology* **53**, 946–55.

Department of Health (1990) *The Community Care Act.* HMSO, London.

Department of Health (1995) *The Carers' Recognition and Service Act.* HMSO, London.

◇ Department of Health (1999) *National Health Service Act.* HMSO, London.

◇ Department of Health (2001a) *Older Peoples National Service Framework.* HMSO, London.

◇ Department of Health (2001b) *The Care Standards Act.* HMSO, London.

◇ Doody RS, Steven JC, Beck C *et al.* (2001) Practice parameter: management of dementia (an evidence based review). Report of the Quality Standards Sub-Committee of the American Academy of Neurology. *Neurology* **56**, 1154–66.

Downs MG (1996) The role of general practice and the primary care team in dementia diagnosis and management. *Int J Geriatr Psychiatry* **11**, 937–42.

Duncan PW, Weiner DK, Chandler J, Studenski S (1990) Functional reach: a new clinical measure of balance. *J Gerontol* **45**, 6.

Eccles M, Clarke J, Livingstone M, Freemantle N, Mason J (1998) North of England Evidence-Based Guidelines development project: guidelines for the primary care management of dementia. *Br Med J* **317**, 802–8.

Ely M, Melzer D, Opit L, Brayne C (1996) Estimating the numbers and characteristics of elderly people with cognitive disability in local populations. *Res Policy Plan* **14**, 13–18.

Ernst RL, Hay JW, Fenn C *et al.* (1997) Cognitive function and the costs of Alzheimer disease: an exploratory study. *Arch Neurol* **54**(6), 687–93.

Everett T, Dennis M, Ricketts E. (1995) *Physiotherapy in Mental Health, a Practical Approach.* Butterworth Heinemann, London.

Fearnley K, McLennan J (1997) *The Right to Know? Sharing the Diagnosis of Dementia.* Alzheimer Scotland – Action on Dementia. Mental Health Foundation, London.

Folstein MF, Folstein SE, McHugh PR (1975) 'Mini-Mental State'. A practical method for grading the cognitive state of patients for the clinician. *J Psychiatr Res* **12**, 189–98.

Forette F, Seux M-L, Staessen JA *et al.* (1998) Prevention of dementia in randomised, double-blind, placebo-controlled systolic hypertension in Europe (Syst-Eur) trial. *Lancet* **352**, 1347–51.

Foster GR, Scott D, Payne S (1999) The use of CAT scanning in dementia: a systematic review. *Int J Tech Assoc Health Care* **15**(2), 406–23.

Fox NC, Cousens S, Scahill R *et al.* (2000) Using serial registered brain magnetic resonance imaging to measure disease progression in Alzheimer's disease: power calculations and estimates of sample size to detect treatment effects. *Arch Neurol* **57**, 339–44.

Furniss L (2000) Effects of a pharmacist's medication review in nursing homes. *Br J Psychiatry* **176**, 563–7.

Gatz M, Reynolds C, Nikolic J *et al.* (1995) An empirical test of telephone screening to identify potential dementia cases. *Int Psychogeriatrics* **7**(3), 429–38.

Getsios D, Caro JJ, Caro G, Ishak K for the AHEAD study group (2001) Assessment of health economics in Alzheimer's disease (AHEAD): galantamine treatment in Canada. *Neurology* **57**, 972–8.

Golding E (1989) *The Middlesex Elderly Assessment of Mental State.* Thames Valley Test Company, Fareham.

Grace J (1994) Alzheimer's disease: your views. *Geriatr Med* **July**, 36–9.

Gray A, Fenn P (1993) Alzheimers's disease: the burden of the illness in England. *Health Trends* **25**, 31–6.

Hagedorn R (1997) *Foundations for Practice in Occupational Therapy*, 2nd edn. Churchill Livingstone, London.

Harding, T. (1997) *A Life Worth Living: the Independence and Inclusion of Older People.* Help the Aged, London.

Harvey R (1998) *Young Onset Dementia: Epidemiology, Clinical Symptoms, Family Burden, Support and Outcome.* Imperial College, London.

◇ Health Advisory Service (HAS 2000) (1998) *Not Because They are Old – an Independent Enquiry into the Care of Older People on Acute Wards in General Hospitals.* NHS Executive, London.

Help the Aged (2000) *Dignity on the Ward: Promoting Excellence in Care, Promoting Practice in Acute Hospital Care for Older People.* The School of Nursing and Midwifery, University of Sheffield.

Henwood M (1998) *Ignored and Invisible: Carers Experience of the NHS.* Carers National Association, London.

Hodkinson HM (1972) Evaluation of a mental test score for assessment of mental impairment in the elderly. *Age Ageing* **1**, 233–8.

Hunter DJ, Wistow G (1990) *Elderly People's Integrated Care System (EPICS): an Organisational Policy and Practice Review.* Nuffield Institute for Health, University of Leeds.

Iliffe S (1994) Evaluation of the use of brief screening instruments for dementia, depression and problem drinking among elderly people in general practice. *Br J Gen Pract* **44**: 503–7.

Iliffe S, Eden A, Downs M, Rae C (1998) The diagnosis and management of dementia in primary care: development, implementation and evaluation of a national training programme. *Ageing Ment Health* **1**, 23–9.

Isaacs B, Neville Y (1975) *The Measurement of Need in Old People*. Scottish Home and Health Department, Edinburgh.

Jeste DV, Caligiuri MP, Paulsen JS *et al.* (1995) Risk of tardive dyskinesia in older patients: a prospective longitudinal study of 266 patients. *Arch Gen Psychiatry* **52**, 756–65.

Jeste DV, Okamoto A, Napolitano J (2000) Low incidence of persistent tardive dyskinesia in elderly patients with dementia treated with risperidone. *Am J Psychiatry* **157**, 1150–5.

Jick H, Zornberg GL, Jick SS *et al.* (2000) Statins and the risk of dementia. *Lancet* **356**, 1627–31.

Jones R (1998) Position statement on specialist old age psychiatry team and nursing and residential care home residents. Good practice principles and potential practice developments. *Psychiatr Bull* **22**, 389–90.

Katz IR, Jeste DV, Mintzer JE *et al.* (1999) Comparison of risperidone and placebo for psychosis and behavioural disturbances associated with dementia: a randomised, double-blind trial. *J Clin Psychiatry* **60**, 107–15.

Katzman R, Brown T, Fuld P *et al.* (1983) Validation of a short orientation-memory-concentration test of cognitive impairment. *Am J Psychiatry* **40**, 734–9.

Kaufer DI, Cummings JL, Christine D *et al.* (1998) Assessing the impact of neuropsychiatric symptoms in Alzheimer's disease: the Neuropsychiatric Inventory Caregiver Distress Scale. *J Am Geriatr Soc* **46**, 210–15.

Kavanagh S, Schneider J, Knapp M *et al.* (1993) Elderly people with cognitive impairment: costing possible changes in the balance of care. *Health Soc Care* **1**, 69–80.

Kavanagh S, Schneider J, Knapp M, *et al.* (1995) Elderly people with dementia: costs, effectiveness, and balance of care. In: Knapp M (ed.), *Economic Evaluation of Mental Health Care*, 125–56. Ashgate Publishing, Hants (England).

Kessler J, Calabrese P, Kalbe E, Berger F (2000) DemTect: a new screening instrument to support the diagnosis of dementia. *Psychology* **26**, 343–7.

Kiresuk TJ, Sherman RE (1968) Goal Attainment Scaling: a general method for evaluating competencies. Community mental health programmes. *Community Ment Health J* **4**, 443–5.

◇ Kitwood T (1997) *Dementia Reconsidered: the Person Comes First*. Open University Press, Buckingham.

Kitwood T (1998) Professional and moral development for care work: some observations on the process. *J Moral Educ* **27**(3), 401–11.

◇ Knopman DS, DeKosky ST, Chui H *et al.* (2001) Practice parameter: diagnosis of dementia (an evidence based review): report of the Quality Standards Committee of the American Academy of Neurology. *Neurology* **56**, 1143–53.

Law M, Baptiste S, Carswell A *et al.* (1998) *Canadian Occupational Performance Measure*, 3rd edn. CAOT Publications ACE, Toronto.

de Lepeleire J, Heyrman J (1994) How do general practitioners diagnose dementia? *Fam Pract* **11**(2), 148–52.

Levin E (1997) *Carers: Problems, Strains and Services.* Oxford University Press, Oxford.

Livingston G, Katona C (2000) How useful are cholinesterase inhibitors in the treatment of Alzheimer's disease? A number needed to treat analysis. *Int J Geriatr Psychiatry* **15**(3), 203–7.

Livingston G, Manela M, Katona C (1997) Cost of community care for older people. *Br J Psychiatry* **171**, 56–69.

Lookinland S, Anson K (1995) Perpetuation of ageist attitudes among present and future health care personnel: implications for elder care. *J Nurs* **21**, 47–56.

Lovestone S, Graham N, Howard R (1997) Guidelines on drug treatment for Alzheimer's disease. *Lancet* **350**, 232–3.

Lundberg C, Johannsson K, Ball K et al. (1997) Dementia and driving: an attempt at consensus. *Alzheimer Dis Assoc Disord* **11**, 28–37.

Mackenzie IRA (2000) Anti-inflammatory drugs and Alzheimer-type pathology in aging. *Neurology* **54**, 732–4.

Maelicke A, Alberquerque EX (1996) New approach to drug therapy in Alzheimer's disease. *Drug Disc Today* **1**(2), 53–9.

Maguire C, Kirby M, Coen R et al. (1996) Family members attitudes toward telling the patient with Alzheimer's disease their diagnosis. *Br Med J* **313**, 529–30.

Mann A, Graham N, Ashby D (1984) Psychiatric illness in residential homes for the elderly: a survey in one London borough. *Age Ageing* **13**, 257–65.

Mayo N (1994) Outcome measures. *Physiother Can* **46**(3), 145–7.

Max W, Webber P, Fox P (1995) Alzheimer's disease: the unpaid burden of caring. *J Aging Health* **7**(2), 179–99.

McCracken M, Boneham M, Copeland J et al. (1997) Prevalence of dementia and depression among elderly people in black and ethnic minorities. *Br J Psychiatry* **171**, 269–73.

McCurry S, Teri L (1997) Advance planning for dementia caregivers. *J Am Geriatr Soc* **45**, 1102–3.

McGeer PL, Schulzer M, McGeer EG (1996) Arthritis and anti-inflammatory agents as possible protective factors for Alzheimer's disease; a review of 17 epidemiologic studies. *Neurology* **47**, 425–32.

McIntosh I, Swanson V, Power K (1997) Stress and dementia management. *Scott Med* **16**, 7–8.

McKeith I, Del Ser T, Spano P et al. (2000) Efficacy of rivastigmine in dementia with Lewy bodies: a randomised, double-blind, placebo-controlled international study. *Lancet* **356**, 2031–6.

McShane R, Keene J, Gedling K et al. (1997) Do neuroleptic drugs hasten cognitive decline in dementia? *Br Med J* **314**, 266–70.

McWilliam, C (1994) A new perspective on threatened autonomy in elderly persons: the disempowering process. *Soc Sci Med* **38**(2), 327–38.

Melzer D, Ely M, Brayne C (1997) Cognitive impairment in elderly people: population based estimate of the future in England, Scotland and Wales. *Br Med J* **315**, 462.

113

Melzer D (1999) Alzheimer's disease and other dementias. In: Stevens A. *et al.* (eds), *Health Care and Needs Assessment: the Epidemiologically Based Needs Assessment Reviews – First Series Update.* Radcliffe Medical Press, Abingdon.

Meyers B (1997) Telling patients with Alzheimer's disease. *Br Med J* **314**, 321–2.

Milne A (1998) *GP Survey.* Tizard Centre, University of Kent.

Mittelman M, Ferris S (1996) A family intervention to delay nursing home placement of patients with Alzheimer's disease. *JAMA* **276**(21), 1725–31.

Mocellin G (1988) Perspective on the principles and practice of occupational therapy. *Br J Occup Ther* **51**(1), 4–7.

Moniz-Cook E, Agar S, Silver M *et al.* (1998) Can staff training reduce behavioural problems in residential care for the elderly mentally ill? *Int J Geriatr Psychiatry* **13**, 149–58.

Mountain G, Godfrey M (1995) *Respite Care Provision for Older People with Dementia: a Review of the Literature.* Nuffield Institute for Health, University of Leeds.

◇ Naidoo M, Bullock R (2001) *An Integrated Care Pathway for Dementia.* Harcourt, London.

◇ National Institute for Clinical Excellence (NICE) (2001) *Clinical and Cost Effectiveness of Donepezil, Rivastigmine and Galantamine for Alzheimer's Disease.* NICE technical appraisal no. 19. Department of Health, London.

Naylor M (1994) Comprehensive discharge planning for the hospitalised elderly. *Ann Intern Med* **120**, 999–1006.

Netten A, Dennett J, Knight J (1998) *Unit Costs of Health and Social Care 1998.* Personal Social Services Research Unit (PSSRU), University of Kent, Canterbury.

Neumann PJ, Kuntz KM, Leon J *et al.* (1999) Health utilities in Alzheimer's disease: a cross-sectional study of patients and caregivers. *Med Care* **37**(1), 27–32.

Nolan M, Cardock K (1996) Assessment: identifying the barriers to good practice. *Health Soc Care Community* **4**(2), 77– 85.

Occupational Therapy Audit (2001) Outcome Measures: COPM and Goal Attainment. Unpublished. Department of Old Age Psychiatry, Swindon.

Occupational Therapy Business Plan (1999/2000) Unpublished. Department of Old Age Psychiatry, Swindon.

O'Connor D, Fertig A (1993) Dementia in general practice: the practical consequences of a more positive approach to diagnosis. *Br J Gen Pract* **43**, 185–8.

O'Connor D, Pollitt P, Roth M *et al.* (1990) Problems reported by relatives in a community study of dementia. *Br J Psychiatry* **156**, 835–41.

Oddy R (1998) *Promoting Mobility for People with Dementia, a Problem Solving Approach.* Age Concern, London.

Pattie AH, Gilleard CJ (1979) *Manual for the Clifton Assessment Procedures for the Elderly (CAPE).* Hodder & Stoughton Educational, Dunton Green, Kent.

Perrin T, May H (2000) *Wellbeing in Dementia: an Occupational Approach for Therapists and Carers.* Churchill Livingstone, London.

◇ Peterson RC, Stevens JC, Ganguli M *et al.* (2001) Practice parameter: early detection of dementia: mild cognitive impairment (an evidence based review):

report of the Quality Standards Committee of the American Academy of Neurology. *Neurology* **56**, 1133–42.

Philp I. (1997) Can a medical and social assessment be combined? *J R Soc Med* **90**(supplement 32), 11–13.

Pinner G (2000) Truth-telling and the diagnosis of dementia. *Br J Psychiatry* **176**, 514–15.

Pollock BG, Mulsant BH, Sweet R *et al.* (1998) An open label pilot study of citalopram for behavioural disturbances of dementia. *Am J Geriatr Psychiatry* **5**(1), 70–8.

Pool J (1999) *The Pool Activity Level (PAL) Instrument: a Practical Resource for Carers of People with Dementia.* Bradford Dementia Group, Jessica Kingsley Publishers, London.

Post SG, Whitehouse P, Binstock RH *et al.* (1997) The clinical introduction of genetic testing for Alzheimer's disease: an ethical perspective. *JAMA* **277**, 832–6.

Rice K, Warner N (1994) Breaking the bad news: what do psychiatrists tell patients with dementia about their illness? *Int J Geriatr Psychiatry* **9**, 467–71.

Ritchie K (1998) Establishing the limits of normal cerebral ageing and senile dementias. *Br J Psychiatry* **173**, 97–101.

Roth M, Mountjoy CQ, Amrein R (1996) Moclobemide in elderly patients with cognitive decline and depression: an international double-blind, placebo-controlled trial. *Br J Psychiatry* **16**(2), 149–57.

◇ Royal Commission on Long Term Care (1999) *With Respect to Old Age: Long Term Care – Rights and Responsibilities.* HMSO, London.

Sano M, Ernesto C, Thomas RG *et al.* (1997) A controlled trial of selegilene, alpha tocopherol, or both as treatment for Alzheimer's disease. *N Engl J Med* **336**, 1216–22.

Satterlee WG, Reams SG, Burns PR *et al.* (1995) A clinical update on olanzapine treatment in schizophrenia and Alzheimer's disease patients. *Psychopharmacol Bull* **31**, 354.

Schenk D, Seubert P, Lieberburg I, Wallace J (2000) B-peptide immunisation; a possible new treatment for Alzheimer's disease. *Arch Neurol* **57**, 934–6.

Scottish Health Service (2000) *Scottish Health Service Costs (year ended 31st March 2000).* Information and Statistics Division. National Health Service in Scotland, Edinburgh.

Sheppard L (1998) *Evaluating The Use of Art Therapy for People with Dementia: a Control Group Study.* Department of Experimental Psychology, University of Sussex, Brighton.

Silveira E, Ebrahim S (1995) Mental health and the status of elderly Bengalis and Somalis in London. *Age Ageing* **24**, 474–80.

Smith R (1994) Validation and reliability of the elderly mobility scale. *Physiotherapy* **80**(11), 774–7.

Social Services Inspectorate (1997) *Older People with Mental Health Problems Living Alone – Anybody's Priority?* SSI, London.

Solomon PR, Hirschoff A, Kelly B *et al.* (1997) A seven minute neurocognitive screening battery highly sensitive to Alzheimer's disease. *Arch Neurol* **55**, 349–55.

Souetre E, Thwaites RM, Yeardley HL (1999) Economic impact of Alzheimer's disease in the United Kingdom. *Br J Psychiatry* **174**, 51–5.

Staton R (ed.) (1996) *Community Care Statistics: Day and Domiciliary Personal Social Services for Adults, Detailed Statistics, England.* Department of Health. HMSO, London.

Stern Y, Tang MX, Albert MS *et al.* (1997) Predicting time to nursing home care and death in individuals with Alzheimer disease. *JAMA* **277**(10), 806–12.

Stewart A, Phillips R, Dempsey G (1998) Pharmacotherapy for people with Alzheimer's disease: a Markov-cycle evaluation of five years' therapy using donepezil. *Int J Geriatr Psychiatry* **13**, 445–53.

Stewart K, Challis D, Carpenter I, Dickinson E (1999) Assessment approaches for older people receiving social care: content and coverage. *Int J Geriatr Psychiatry* **14**, 147–56.

Street JS, Clark WS, Gannon KS *et al.* (2000) Olanzapine treatment of psychotic and behavioural symptoms in patients with Alzheimer disease in nursing care facilities. *Arch Gen Psychiatry* **57**, 968–76.

Svanberg R, Stirling E (1997) The process of care management with people with dementia. *Health Soc Care Community* **5**(2), 134–46.

Tang M-X, Jacobs D, Stern Y *et al.* (1996) Effect of oestrogen during menopause on risk of Alzheimer's disease. *Lancet* **348**, 429–32.

Tariot P, Solomon PR, Morris J *et al.* (2000) A 5-month, randomised, placebo-controlled trial of galantamine in AD. *Neurology* **54**, 2269–76.

Teri L (1999) Effects of caregiver training and behavioural strategies in Alzheimer's disease. In: Iqbal K (ed.), *Alzheimer's Disease and Related Disorders.* Wiley, Chichester.

Tinetti ME, Williams TF, Mayewski R (1986) Fall risk index for elderly patients based on number of chronic disabilities. *Am J Med* **80**, 429–34.

Trieman N, Wills N (1996) The psychogeriatric population: in transition from hospital to community based services. In: Leff J (ed.), *Care in the Community: Illusion or Reality.* Wiley, Chichester.

Tullis A, Nicol M (1999) A systematic review of the evidence for the value of functional assessment of older people with dementia. *Br J Occup Ther* **62**(12), 554–64.

Twigg J (ed.) (1992) *Carers: Research and Practice.* HMSO, London.

van Crevel H, van Gool WA, Waistra GJM (1999) Early diagnosis of dementia. Which tests are indicated? What are their costs? *J Neurol* **246**, 73–8.

Wald J (1983) Alzheimer's disease – and the role of art therapy in its treatment. *Am J Art Ther* **22**, 57–64.

Wald J (1984) The graphic representation of regression in an Alzheimer's disease patient. *Arts Psychother* **11**, 165–75.

Wald J (1986) Art therapy for patients with dementing illnesses. *Clin Geneol* **14**(3), 29–40.

Waldemar G, Dubois B, Emre M *et al.* (2000) Diagnosis and management of Alzheimer's disease and other disorders associated with dementia. The role of neurologists in Europe. *Eur J Neurol* **7**(2), 133–44.

Waller D, Dally T (1992) Art therapy: a theoretical perspective. In: Waller D, Gilroy A (eds), *Art Therapy: a Handbook.* Open University Press, Buckingham.

Warchol K (2000) The challenge of dementia care. *OT Pract* **Nov 6**, 15–19.

Warren AF (1999) An evaluation of the Canadian Occupational Performance Measure and the factors that influence its use by occupational therapists within mental health practice. Unpublished MSc Occupational Therapy Dissertation, University of Wales, College of Medicine.

Wilkinson P (1997) Cognitive therapy with older people. *Age Ageing* **26**, 53–8.

Wimo A, Krakau L, Mattson B, Nelvig A (1994) The impact of cognitive decline on the costs of dementia care. *Int J Geriatr Psychiatry* **9**, 479–89.

Wolfson C, Moride Y, Perrault A *et al.* (2000) *Drug Treatments for Alzheimer's Disease. II. A Review of Outcome Measures in Clinical Trials.* Canadian Coordinating office for Health Technology Assessment (CCOHTA), Ottawa.

World Health Organization (1992) *The ICD-10 Classification of Mental and Behavioural Disorders.* WHO, Geneva.

World Health Organization (1998) Organization of care in psychiatry of the elderly – a technical consensus statement. WHO/WPA. *Aging Ment Health* **2**(3), 246–52.

Wright N, Lindesay J (1995) A survey of memory clinics in the British Isles. *Int J Geriatr Psychiatry* **10**, 379–85.

FURTHER ESSENTIAL READING

Briggs K, Askham J (1999) *The Needs of People with Dementia and Those who Care for Them: a Review of the Literature.* Alzheimer's Society, London.
Burns A, Lawlor B, Craig S. (1999) *Assessment Scales in Old Age Psychiatry.* Martin Dunitz, London.
Burns A, Dening T, Lawlor B (2001) *Clinical Guidelines in Old Age Psychiatry.* Martin Dunitz, London.
Department of Health (1997) *A Handbook on the Mental Health of Older People.* HMSO, London.
Department of Health (1997) *Better Services for Vulnerable People.* EL (97) 62, CI (97) 24.
Department of Health (1998) *Partnership in Action.* HMSO, London.
Department of Health (1998) *Modernising Social Services.* The Stationery Office, London.
Department of Health (2000) *The NHS Plan: a Plan for Investment. A Plan for Reform.* HMSO, London.
Health Advisory Service (1999) *Standards for Health and Social Care Services for Older People.* Pavillion, Brighton.
Help the Aged (1997) *A Life Worth Living.* Help the Aged, London.
Palmer, C. (1999) *EBB Evidence Based Briefing: Dementia.* Gaskell, London.
Royal College of Psychiatrists and Royal College of Physicians (1998) *The Care of Older People with Mental Illness: Specialist Services and Medical Training.* Royal Colleges, London.

INDEX

goal attainment framework 51
graduates to service 87–8

health economic assessment 39–40
health economic modelling 40–2
health trusts 1
heritability of dementias 76–7
Huntington's disease 56, 76
hypertension, dementia risk factor 84
hypothalamic atrophy 105

illness duration 41
imaging 17, 18, 105
independence, maximising 63
institutionalisation
  delay 65
  psychiatric disorders 79
  see also care home sector; nursing
    home care
instruments for care team 26, 27–30, 31
integrated care
  pathway 12
  programme approach 35
intermediate care 73, 84
interventions, economic value 39

jabadao 58–9

language see speech and language
    therapy (SALT)
leisure, occupational therapy 51
Lewy body dementia 67, 79
  drug actions 82
liaison services 84–5
lorazepam 82

magnetic resonance imaging (MRI) 105
management policy 31
memory assessment process 38
Memory Clinic Association (UK) 22
memory clinics 14, 18, 20–3
  commissioning 22–3
  early-stage patients 38–9
  GP enthusiasts 69
  occupational therapy 51
  referral to speech and language therapy
    46
  services 21
  standardisation 21–2
  trigger questions 39
  types 20
mental health trusts 94

mental illness, late-onset 3, 88
Middlesex Elderly Assessment of Mental
    State (MEAMS) 11
Mini-Mental State Examination (MMSE) 10
moclobemide 81
mood stabilisers 82
multidisciplinary teams 4, 62
  assessment 85
  occupational therapists 49
  ongoing care 90

National Institute for Clinical Excellence
    (NICE) 4
  antipsychotics 68, 81
  cholinesterase inhibitor endorsement
    63, 66–8
  funding allocation 21
  guidance 8, 21
National Service Framework (NSF) for
    older people 45, 47, 90, 91
  impact on old age psychiatry/dementia
    services 92
  recommendations 67
  standard 91
neglect, passive 86
neuroleptics 86
neurology 91
neuropsychological testing 21–2
  psychologists 59
neuropsychology 18
  resource availability 17
nicotinic receptors
  changes 105
  modulating effects of galantamine 64
nitrazepam 82
non-steroidal anti-inflammatory drugs
    (NSAIDs) protective effect 105
nurse prescribing 81, 87, 106
nurses, specialist 106
nursing home care 66
  costs 41
  occupational therapy 51
  resources 87
  services 85–7
  see also care home sector;
    institutionalisation

occupational therapy 47–51, 61
  assessment 49–50
  development in dementia services
    48–9
  goal attainment framework 51

123

risk assessment
  forms *32–3*
  policy 31
risperidone 81, *82*
rivastigmine 82
Royal College of Speech and Language
  Therapists (RCSLT) 44, 45

7-minute screen 10
schizophrenia 88
secondary care, information requested
  14–15
service provision
  liaison services 84–5
  modernising 78–89
shared care 106
  protocols 69
sleep disturbance 81–2
social isolation 54
social services 16, 91
  involvement 66
speech and language therapy (SALT)
  44–7, *61*
  assessment 45–6
  intervention 46
  role 45–6
  service provision 45

statins protective effect 105
swallowing disorders 44, 46–7

tacrine *82*
temazepam 82
thioridazine 82
trainees 20
treatment 63–70
  development 106
  general practitioner roles 68–70
  symptomatic 8, 65
  see also cholinesterase inhibitors
tricyclic antidepressants, contraindication
  81

valproate 82
vitamin E 107
voluntary sector 75

waiting lists 14, 22, 74
World Health Organisation/World
  Psychiatric Association (WHO/WPA)
  consensus guidelines 99

younger people with dementia 51, 76–7
  services 88

zoplicone 82